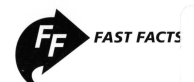
FAST FACTS

M000308007

Digital Medicine – Measurement

Andrea Coravos
Elektra Labs, Harvard-MIT Center for Regulatory Science, and The Digital Medicine Society, Boston, MA, USA

Jennifer C Goldsack
The Digital Medicine Society, Boston, MA, USA

Daniel R Karlin
The Digital Medicine Society, Boston, MA, HealthMode, New York, NY, and Tufts University School of Medicine, Boston, MA, USA

Camille Nebeker
Department of Family Medicine and Public Health, and Center for Wireless and Population Health Systems, School of Medicine, University of California, San Diego, La Jolla, CA, USA

Eric Perakslis
Duke Forge, Durham, NC, and Harvard Medical School, Boston, MA, USA

Noah Zimmerman
Tempus Labs Inc., Chicago, IL, USA

M Kelley Erb
Digital and Quantitative Medicine, Biogen Inc., Cambridge, MA, USA

Declaration of Independence
This book is as balanced and as practical as we can make it.
Ideas for improvement are always welcome: fastfacts@karger.com

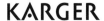
KARGER

Fast Facts: Digital Medicine – Measurement
First published as Coravos A, Goldsack JC, Karlin DR et al. Digital medicine: a primer on measurement. *Digit Biomark* 2019;3:31–71. doi: 10.1159/000500413.

S. Karger Publishers Ltd, Elizabeth House, Queen Street, Abingdon, Oxford OX14 3LN, UK
Tel: +44 (0)1235 523233

Book orders can be placed by telephone or email, or via the website.
Please telephone +41 61 306 1440 or email orders@karger.com
To order via the website, please go to karger.com
Fast Facts is a trademark of S. Karger Publishers Ltd.

A CIP record for this title is available from the British Library.

ISBN 978-3-318-06707-1

Coravos A (Andrea)
Fast Facts: Digital Medicine – Measurement/
Andrea Coravos, Jennifer C Goldsack, Daniel R Karlin, Camille Nebeker, Eric Perakslis, Noah Zimmerman, M Kelley Erb

Illustrations by Cognitive Media Ltd.
Typesetting by Thomas Bohm, User Design, Illustration and Typesetting, UK.
Printed in the UK with Xpedient Print.

Acknowledgments

For refinement of ideas, frameworks and terms relating to digital medicine, the authors gratefully acknowledge Adam Conner-Simons, Beau Woods, Jessie Bakker and Emily Singer. They also acknowledge the team at COGNI+IVE (wearecognitive.com) for bringing their ideas to life as illustrations and Pfizer Inc. for funding the illustrations.

Glossary

AI: Artificial intelligence

Analytic validation: The process of ensuring that the algorithm processing the data is reporting the measure of interest

Belmont Report: 1979 report that describes three guiding principles of ethical biomedical and behavioral research: respect for persons, beneficence and justice

Biomarker: A defined characteristic that is measured as an indicator of normal biological processes, pathogenic processes or responses to an exposure or intervention

CBCT: Community-based clinical trial, a study conducted primarily through primary-care physicians rather than academic research facilities

CBER: US Food and Drug Administration Center for Biologics Evaluation and Research

CCPA: California Consumer Privacy Act, implemented in 2020; gives consumers control over their data and requires that companies explain what they collect and how they use and share data

CDER: US Food and Drug Administration Center for Drug Evaluation and Research

CDRH: US Food and Drug Administration Center for Devices and Radiological Health

CDS: Clinical decision support

CGM: Continuous glucose monitor

Clinical outcome: A measurable characteristic that describes or reflects how an individual feels, functions or survives

ClinRO: Clinician-reported outcome, a measurement based on a report that comes from a trained healthcare professional after observation of a patient's health condition

Clinical validation: Process of ensuring the assessment acceptably reflects the concept of interest

COA: Clinical outcome assessment

Combination product: A medical product composed of any combination of: a drug and a device; a biological product and a device; a drug and a biological product; or a drug, device and a biological product

Context of use: Regulatory term describing how a tool is used and where it is applied

CORE initiative: Connected and Open Research Ethics initiative, a learning 'ethics' resource developed to support the digital medicine research community

CTTI: Clinical Trials Transformation Initiative, a public–private partnership co-founded by Duke University and the US Food and Drug Administration

Cures Act: The 21st Century Cures Act, which was signed into US law on 13 December 2016 and which intended to modernize the US healthcare system, recognizing the central roles of technology and science; among other impacts, it amended the definition of device in the Food, Drug, and Cosmetic Act to exclude certain software functions

CVE: Common Vulnerabilities and Exposures program, operated by MITRE; identifies and catalogs vulnerabilities in software and firmware into a free dictionary

CWG: Cybersecurity Working Group

DCT: Decentralized clinical trial; to determine the level of decentralization, consider where the data are captured (i.e. near the patient?) and how they are captured (e.g. manually?)

DDT: Drug Development Tool, a US Food and Drug Administration qualification program

DICE: Division of Industry and Consumer Education at the US Food and Drug Administration

Digital intervention products: Digital therapeutics and connected implantables (e.g. an insulin pump)

Digital measurement products: Include digital biomarkers, electronic clinical outcome assessments and digital tools that measure adherence and safety

Digital medicine: A field that uses technologies as tools for measurement and intervention in the service of human health

DiMe: The Digital Medicine Society

DMD: Duchenne's muscular dystrophy

Ecological validity: How test performance predicts behavior in a real-world setting

EHR: Electronic health record

EKG: Electrocardiogram

ELSI: Ethical, legal and social implications

EMA: European Medicines Agency

Endpoint: A precisely defined variable intended to reflect an outcome of interest that is statistically analyzed to address a particular research question

Enforcement discretion: Occurs when the US Food and Drug Administration determines that a product is a device but chooses not to regulate it

EU: European Union

EULA: End user license agreement

FDA: US Food and Drug Administration

GDPR: General Data Protection Regulations, which took effect in the European Union (EU) in 2018 and aim to safeguard EU citizens' data privacy

HHS: US Department of Health and Human Services

HOCMD: Hippocratic Oath for Connected Medical Devices, which outlines five guiding security and ethical principles for manufacturers, organizations and individuals delivering care through connected medical devices

HSCC: Health Sector Coordinating Council

ICT: Information and communication technologies

IMDRF: International Medical Device Regulators Forum

IoB: Internet of Bodies, a network of smart devices attached to or inside human bodies

IoT: Internet of Things

IRB: Institutional review board

Legacy standard: Term for widely used existing standard where a new and better standard has been developed, preferred to 'gold standard'

MDDT: Medical device development tool

MMA: Mobile medical application

Menlo Report: Adapted the ethical principles of the Belmont Report to information and communication technologies, adding a fourth principle, that of respect for the law and public interest

MS: Multiple sclerosis

Multimodal data: Collected from different sources of clinical data (e.g. sensors, questionnaires, lab tests)

NIH: National Institutes of Health

NIST: National Institute of Standards and Technology

ObsRO: Observer-reported outcome, assessment of how a person feels or functions in daily life made by non-expert third party

OHRP: Federal Office for Human Research Protections

PDS: Patient decision support

PDURS: Prescription drug-use-related software, developed for use with prescription drugs (e.g. tracking drug ingestion)

PerfO: Performance outcome, a measurement based on standardized task(s) performed by a patient that is administered and evaluated by an appropriately trained individual or is independently completed

PHI: Personal health information

PII: Personally identifiable information

PMA: Premarket approval

PMDA: Pharmaceuticals and Medical Device Agency

Predicate: Legally marketed medical device with which a new product would claim equivalence

PRO: Patient-reported outcome, self-assessment of how a person feels or functions in daily life reported without modification or interpretation

RCT: Randomized controlled trial

REB: Research ethics board

SaMD: Software as a medical device

SBOM: Software bill of materials, a list of components in a given piece of software

Security: The application of protections and management of risk posed by cyber threats

ToS: Terms of service

V&V: Verification and validation

Validation: Process of ensuring the tool is meeting its intended use by generating objective data that accurately represent the concept of interest; answers the question 'did I build the right tool?'

Verification: Assessment of sensor accuracy, precision, consistency and/or uniformity; answers the question 'did I make the tool right?'

White hat hacker: Performs ethical hacking of a network and uses coordinated disclosure to the network owner when vulnerabilities are found

Introduction

Digital medicine products hold great promise to improve medical measurement, diagnosis and treatment. While many industries have embraced digital disruption, the healthcare industry has yet to experience the improvements in outcomes, access and cost-effectiveness long promised by the digital revolution. Healthcare lags behind other industries in part because of the regulatory environment, which tends to slow progress as health authorities strive to minimize adverse outcomes.

Developing effective digital medicine tools is an intensive and challenging process that requires the interdisciplinary efforts of a wide range of experts, from engineers and ethicists to payers and providers. Many of the challenges are compounded by the multidisciplinary nature of this field. The advancement of digital medicine stalls when constituent experts speak different languages and have different standards, experiences and expectations.

The Digital Medicine Society (DiMe), the professional society for practitioners of digital medicine, exists to address these challenges.[1] We believe that effective communication is essential for turning scientific discoveries into commercial products. Having unclear definitions and inconsistent terminology hinders our abilities to evaluate scientific evidence and, ultimately, develop successful medical products. Our goals with this book are to:

- promote effective collaboration among different stakeholders by providing a common framework of language and ideas within which to collaborate
- support the advancement of measurement in digital medicine by clarifying core concepts and terms.

To achieve these goals, we have synthesized the basics of clinical medicine, medical research, regulation and ethics into an accessible and digestible form and, by clarifying core concepts and terms, we aim to drive the field forward.

Fast Facts: Digital Medicine – Measurement focuses specifically on measurement in digital medicine, a foundational component underpinning the decentralization and democratization of clinical care and clinical trials using digital tools. We also explicate relationships between digital measurement in research and digital measurement in clinical care. Though these are interrelated concepts, and much technology moves fluidly between research and care, we have chosen to focus on research as this seems to be a logical sequence. The ability to demonstrate reliability and meaningfulness for clinical trials, whether clinic based or otherwise, will ultimately translate into clinical use. Although the research space is fragmented, it is far more cohesive and unitary than clinical care. We believe that effecting changes in practice across the research domain in a timely manner is a feasible goal that will benefit patient care both through the translation of new technology and the creation and approval of novel treatments. While our treatment of clinical care may seem sparse, we do attempt to cover a breadth of applicable examples.

This book has been written with a wide readership in mind:

- technology experts, including software engineers, designers, data scientists, security researchers and product managers who want to deepen their healthcare knowledge
- academic researchers and industry sponsors of clinical trials who need to facilitate internal discussions across teams (e.g. data science teams working with protocol designers in the translational medicine teams)
- clinicians, who will be increasingly exposed to digital medicine in their practice
- members of the public who, we believe, will drive more of their own healthcare as the practice of medicine becomes more personalized and consumer-oriented.

As leaders in our field have stated before us, if we are successful in accelerating the advancement of digital medicine, then soon, it will just be part of 'medicine'.[2] We share the same vision for the future.

Using this book

Important terms or phrases for the field are summarized in the glossary. Where possible, we reference existing definitions. Where we found conflicting definitions, we propose a revised definition. We hope that standardizing terminology will help unify and advance the field. We also recognize that these definitions will evolve over time. Borrowing from the success of our colleagues in cancer immunotherapy, and research in emergency medicine, we have distilled key clinical ontologies and frameworks into cartoon illustrations.[3,4]

Where regulatory issues are addressed, this book is biased toward US pathways and requirements. It is noteworthy that, as the field of medicine evolves in the digital era, there is limited harmonization in approaches across regulatory regions. Future books in this series on Digital Medicine will provide a global perspective on regulatory requirements.

We have organized the book as follows.

- Chapters 1 and 2 provide an overview of digital medicine, focusing on the software and algorithms that are being used to measure individuals' health and intervene to improve their condition.
- Chapters 3–6 are written for readers newer to the ethical, legal/regulatory and social implications (ELSI) associated with health research and healthcare; we provide an overview of 'clinical research' versus routine 'clinical care' and the considerations as a product goes to market.
- Chapters 7–9 introduce terms that classify types of digital measurements, such as digital biomarkers and electronic clinical outcome assessments. They also describe how to think through developing a digital measure for use in a clinical trial setting versus clinical care – and important considerations to ensure the measures are trustworthy, such as the concepts of verification and validation.
- Chapter 10 describes our collective responsibilities as we intentionally build the future of digital medicine.

References

1. The Digital Medicine Society (DiMe). *The Digital Medicine Society*, 2019. www.dimesociety.org, last accessed 8 September 2019.

2. Steinhubl SR, Topol EJ. Digital medicine, on its way to being just plain medicine. *npj Digit Med* 2018;1:20175.

3. Canavan N. Cartoons offer a peek into cancer immunotherapy — and scientists' minds. *STAT*, 2018. www.statnews.com/2018/10/17/cancer-immunotherapy-scientists-cartoons, last accessed 30 July 2019.

4. Delp C, Jones J. Communicating information to patients: the use of cartoon illustrations to improve comprehension of instructions. *Acad Emerg Med* 1996;3:264–70.

1   What is digital medicine?

Digital medicine describes a field concerned with the use of technologies as tools for measurement and intervention in the service of human health. Digital medicine products are driven by high-quality hardware and software products that support health research and the practice of medicine broadly, including treatment, recovery, disease prevention and health promotion for individuals and across populations (Figure 1.1).

Role of products

Digital medicine products can be used independently or in concert with pharmaceuticals, biologics, devices or other products to optimize patient care and health outcomes. Patients and healthcare providers are empowered with intelligent and accessible tools to address a wide range of conditions through high-quality, safe and effective measurements and data-driven interventions. Digital products are also used in health research to develop knowledge of the fundamental determinants of health and illness by examining biological, environmental and lifestyle factors. In observational and interventional research, digital technologies are increasingly used in the prevention and treatment of disease and to support health promotion.

As a discipline, digital medicine encapsulates both broad professional expertise and responsibilities concerning the use of these digital tools. Digital medicine focuses on evidence generation to support the use of these technologies. Measurement products include digital biomarkers (e.g. using a vocal biomarker to track changes in tremor for a Parkinson's patient), electronic clinical outcome assessments (e.g. an electronic patient-reported outcome survey) and tools that measure adherence and safety (e.g. a wearable sensor that tracks falls and smart mirrors for passive monitoring in the home).[1]

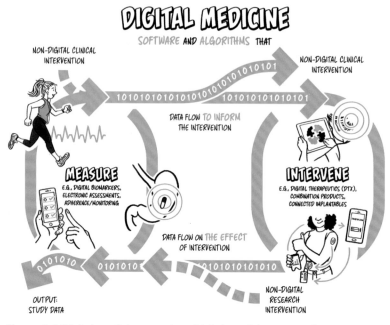

Figure 1.1 Digital medicine overview. Digital medicine uses software and algorithmically driven products to measure or intervene to improve human health.

Intervention products include digital therapeutics and connected implantables (e.g. an insulin pump). Digital therapeutics deliver evidence-based therapeutic interventions to patients that are driven by high-quality software programs to prevent, manage or treat a medical disorder or disease. They are used independently or in concert with medications, devices or other therapies to optimize patient care and health outcomes.[2] Digital intervention products are not the primary focus of this book, however.

Combination products both measure and intervene. For example, continuous glucose monitors (CGMs) for people with diabetes share data from a patient automatically with their doctor's office using a companion app. The level of human involvement may vary in the cycle between measurement and intervention – for example, when a doctor diagnoses an abnormal heart condition from an electrocardiogram (EKG) reading off a smartphone. Over time, this cycle may become more of a closed loop, with less need for human intervention in response to routine changes. The development of the 'artificial pancreas' has combined the CGM with an insulin pump and a computer-controlled algorithm that allows the system to automatically adjust the delivery of insulin to reduce high blood glucose levels (hyperglycemia) and minimize the incidence of low blood glucose (hypoglycemia).[3]

Digital health

Similar to the way in which 'wellness' products differ from those used in medicine, 'digital health' differs from digital medicine. We use 'digital health' to describe products that consumers use to measure physical activity or sleep quality – things that might influence their personal wellbeing. Digital health products may include apps or wearable sensors (e.g. Fitbit, Oura ring). Digital health products are intended to be consumer-facing rather than used in clinical care; they often do not produce the evidence necessary to support medical use.

There are times when it may be appropriate to use consumer-grade tools for measurement in clinical research. For example, using an accelerometer manufactured for the consumer market to measure physical activity among research participants enrolled in a clinical trial is common. However, this would require a reasonable body of evidence to support this use (see chapter 9 on verification and validation).

Digital medicine product manufacturers commit to undergo rigorous randomized controlled clinical studies for their products. Unlike digital health products, digital medicine products demonstrate success in clinical trials.[4] In this book, we outline digital products that measure and intervene in all areas of the practice of medicine, extending to and including behavioral health, public health and population health management.

Usage. We have decided not to use the term 'digital health'. While it is one of the buzziest catchphrases in the industry today, it has been so broadly used and misinterpreted that it has no real meaning. Instead, we use **digital medicine** as the term to describe evidence-based digital products that measure and intervene, including those intended for health promotion and disease prevention. Digital medicine products are evidence-based tools that support health research and the practice of medicine. Digital medicine describes this broad, evidence-based field and does not refer to the narrow use of the term 'medicine', which is sometimes interpreted as the drug ('medicine') that is administered to the patient.

Algorithms, machine learning and artificial intelligence

The recent explosion of machine learning and artificial intelligence methods, driven in large part by the availability of massive datasets and inexpensive computation, has played an important role in enabling digital medicine products.[5] Whereas traditional health measures represent a snapshot in time – a lab value, a diagnostic image, a blood pressure reading or a note in a medical record – connected digital devices offer a longitudinal and highly personalized window into human health.

A key component of these systems is the transformation of raw physiological or environmental signals into health indicators that can be used to monitor and predict aspects of health and disease. These data (e.g. from a sensor) are processed, transformed and used to build computational models with output that represents the health indicators of interest. Computational approaches range from simple statistical models like linear regression, to signal processing methods like the Fourier transform, to time series analyses like additive regression models, or machine learning methods like support vector machines or convolutional neural networks.

For example, an algorithm is required to transform the raw data from a three-axis accelerometer into the more widely usable health indicator of step counts. There are a variety of different approaches to this task, yielding a variety of different performance characteristics.[6] Importantly, the more examples of real-world walking that the algorithm has access to – by people of different shapes and sizes, under different conditions – the greater the opportunity to improve the accuracy of the model.

Digital measurements in medicine today

Some digital measurements are already well established in routine clinical care – ambulatory EKG monitoring, for example, is used to detect arrhythmias in cardiac patients.[7] Similarly, remotely monitoring patients with implanted heart devices allows doctors to better follow their cardiac patients, detecting abnormal heart rhythms and problems with the device sooner.

Digital measures are also used in clinical research to better monitor patients and more efficiently assess safety and efficacy. For example, in-hospital ambulatory cardiac monitoring has existed for many years, enabling real-time monitoring of EKG signals. Similarly, portable EKG technologies have also existed; these recorded signals for later analysis. The digital medicine solutions for cardiac monitoring include non-obtrusive patch-based cardiac monitors that may be worn for days at a time, while ambulatory and remote from the hospital, and which send real-time signals.

Across therapeutic areas and technologies, digital medicine solutions can solve weaknesses of existing solutions, and can come to market with more patient-friendly packages. Some examples of products used in clinical care are described below.

Recovery, performance and treatment selection. In patients recovering from orthopedic surgery, app-enabled wearable sensors are increasingly being used during rehabilitation. Digital measurements, such as range of motion and step count, allow remote monitoring of a patient's progress. More sophisticated measurements can monitor in real-time if a patient is doing their rehab exercises.

Real-time safety monitoring. Digital fall detection systems allow remote monitoring of elderly and frail individuals. Such monitoring often relies on wearable sensors, cameras, motion sensors, microphones and/or floor sensors.

Treatment adherence. One of the thorniest problems in routine clinical care can now be measured under limited circumstances. An ingestible sensor embedded in a medication is available to monitor when a pill is taken. When the sensor interacts with stomach acid, it transmits to a patch sensor worn over the abdomen. Abilify MyCite is the only drug combined with a digital ingestion tracking system to be approved in the US, though it was approved with no new label claims and was received skeptically by the psychiatric community.[8,9] Other innovations, like 'smart packs', integrate sensors into the packaging of medicines to record when the drug was administered and deliver automatic reminders to take a medication.

Multimodal data integration. By combining remotely captured data into electronic medical records (EMRs), personal health records, patient portals and clinical data repositories, innovators hope to improve clinical decision-making and support data-driven medicine.[10]

Potential applications in clinical research include the following.
- Data collected from remote sensors could be used as a novel endpoint for hard-to-measure conditions like Parkinson's.[11,12]
- Digital measures are being used to assess medication adherence in clinical trials using smart blister packages for investigational drugs.
- Continuous digital measures may allow for the detection of safety events that would otherwise go unrecorded – for example, a wearable cardiac monitor can help reveal arrhythmia in research participants during trials of stimulant use in people with attention deficit hyperactivity disorder (ADHD).
- Digital measures may enable more objective and precise screening for inclusion/exclusion in a clinical trial, which could expand the pool of eligible research participants, increase diversity of a trial population and decrease attrition between evaluation and enrollment by returning information to researchers faster.
- Digital measures may inform better decisions about whether to progress a drug from early phase trials to later, larger and more costly trials. These are known as 'go/no go' decisions. Digital measures may be particularly important to inform these decisions where current measures are subjective and/or where there is a high failure rate. For example, in Alzheimer's disease, digital cognitive assessments that afford more sensitive and frequent monitoring, but are not endorsed by health authorities yet, could enable better decision-making about which treatments to advance to the next phase of clinical development (Box 1.1).[13]

Articles reviewing current and prospective wearable technologies and their progress toward clinical application and the use of medical technology in the home provide additional examples of measurement in digital medicine.[7,15]

BOX 1.1

An example of how digital measures can improve screening in clinical trials

In oncology trials, one key inclusion criterion is performance status, an assessment of the extent to which potential participants' disease affects their ability to do activities of daily life, which is considered subjective and difficult to assess accurately.[14] A real-time digital measurement of performance status could reduce the variability of this assessment in trials and help ensure enrollment of the intended patient as a research participant.

In summary, the field of digital medicine applies the same rigor to the selection, development or use of digital technology for measurement and intervention that is applied to other areas of medicine. In chapters 3–6, we outline security, ethical, legal and regulatory considerations when adopting digital medicine technologies in clinical research and routine care (Figure 1.2).

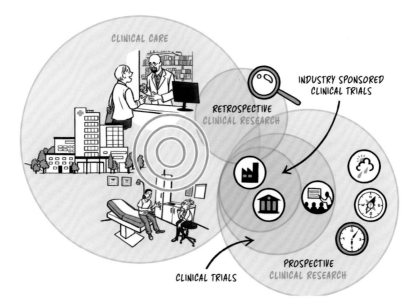

Figure 1.2 The clinical landscape. The healthcare landscape can be broadly split into premarket clinical research and postmarket clinical care.

Key points – what is digital medicine?

- Digital medicine is an emerging medical and scientific discipline concerned with the application of software and hardware to health through cycles of innovation and development of research-based evidence.
- Digital medicine products can be used for measurement and/or treatment, and in combination with existing diagnostics and therapeutics.
- Measurement using digital products may enable more continuous, more precise and less biased information than traditional means of measurement in medicine.
- These measurement advantages are applicable in clinical care and in the conduct of clinical research, where such measurements can be used as clinical endpoints or for other measurement and monitoring purposes such as establishing eligibility for a trial or detecting adverse effects of a treatment under study.

References

1. Miotto R, Danieletto M, Scelza JR, Kidd BA, Dudley JT. Reflecting health: smart mirrors for personalized medicine. *npj Digit Med* 2018;1:62.

2. Digital Therapeutics Alliance. *Digital Therapeutics: Combining Technology and Evidence-based Medicine To Transform Personalized Patient Care*, 2018. www.dtxalliance. org/wp-content/uploads/2018/09/ DTA-Report_DTx-Industry-Foundations.pdf, last accessed 30 July 2019.

3. Linebaugh K. Citizen hackers tinker with medical devices. *Wall Street Journal*, 2014. www.wsj. com/articles/citizen-hackers-concoct-upgrades-for-medical-devices-1411762843?tesla=y, last accessed 30 July 2019.

4. Coravos A. The doctor prescribes video games and virtual reality rehab. *Wired*, 2018. www.wired.com/story/ prescription-video-games-and-vr-rehab/, last accessed 30 July 2019.

5. Esteva A, Robicquet A, Ramsundar B et al. A guide to deep learning in healthcare. *Nat Med* 2019;25:24–9.

6. Kooiman TJ, Dontje ML, Sprenger SR et al. Reliability and validity of ten consumer activity trackers. *BMC Sports Sci Med Rehabil* 2015;7:24.

7. Dunn J, Runge R, Snyder M. Wearables and the medical revolution. *Per Med* 2018;15:429–48.

8. US Food and Drug Administration. *FDA Approves Pill with Sensor that Digitally Tracks if Patients have Ingested their Medication*, 2017. www.fda.gov/newsevents/newsroom/ pressannouncements/ucm584933. htm, last accessed 30 July 2019.

9. Rosenbaum L. Swallowing a spy — the potential uses of digital adherence monitoring. *N Engl J Med* 2017;378:101–3.

10. Shameer K, Badgeley MA, Miotto R et al. Translational bioinformatics in the era of real-time biomedical, health care and wellness data streams. *Brief Bioinform* 2017; 18:105–24.

11. Clinical Trials Transformation Initiative. *CTTI Recommendations: Developing Novel Endpoints Generated by Mobile Technologies For Use in Clinical Trials*, 2017. www.ctti-clinicaltrials.org/files/ novelendpoints-recs.pdf, last accessed 30 July 2019.

12. Izmailova ES, Wagner JA, Perakslis ED. Wearable devices in clinical trials: hype and hypothesis. *Clin Pharmacol Ther* 2018;104:42–52.

13. Fillit HM. FDA removes an unnecessary barrier to testing Alzheimer's drugs. *STAT*, 2018. www.statnews.com/2018/03/05/alzheimers-disease-drugs-fda/, last accessed 30 July 2019.

14. Kosov M, Kolesnik V, Riefler J, Belotserkovskiy M. Implication of Murphy's Law in clinical trials. *J Neoplasm* 2017;2:13.

15. Ten Haken I, Ben Allouch S, van Harten WH. The use of advanced medical technologies at home: a systematic review of the literature. *BMC Public Health* 2018;18:284.

2 Where does digital medicine fit?

Within the clinical space

Clinical care is familiar to most readers from their own experiences with doctors, hospitals and other parts of the healthcare system. Historically, its primary purpose has been to address health problems, and it has long been grounded in the interaction between a patient and a healthcare provider. There has been varying progression of healthcare activities toward preventive care and the maintenance of wellness. With the introduction of connected technologies, there have also been attempts to move healthcare activities into the home, decreasing the need for face-to-face interactions with providers. Clinical care activities include a wide range of diagnostic and treatment processes and procedures, such as:

- real-time monitoring – for example, with continuous blood glucose sensors
- tools to support medical adherence, such as smart apps and pill dispensers
- physical rehabilitation tools, such as digital activity trackers.

Clinical research may include some of the same activities as clinical care, but the primary purpose of clinical research is to develop a better understanding of factors influencing health and illness in people. The federal regulations define research as a 'systematic investigation, including research development, testing and evaluation, designed to develop or contribute to generalizable knowledge'.[1] When a person (e.g. patient or healthy individual) volunteers to enroll in clinical research, they are called a research participant. There are rules and guidance that must be followed when conducting clinical research to make sure that research participants are protected from undue risks of harm. Clinical research comes in two broad subsets.

- In **interventional studies**, participants receive some form of treatment, education or support (Box 2.1). Clinical trials are a subset of interventional studies designed to evaluate the safety and efficacy of an intervention.
- In **non-interventional studies**, participants do not receive an intervention. Non-interventional studies include observational, exploratory, survey, case–control, cohort and correlational studies. Computational studies that use existing data sources to build predictive models fall into this category.

BOX 2.1

Interventional studies

In interventional studies, participants are typically randomized at enrollment to either receive the investigational intervention (experimental arm) or the placebo/current standard of care (control arm). Comparing how participants in these two groups respond allows us to understand the safety and efficacy of the intervention.

Outside the clinic walls

Like any other medical tool, at-home monitoring technologies need to prove their worth. Developers, working with researchers and other experts, must demonstrate that these tools produce clinically meaningful information that leads to clinically meaningful improvements in care, processes and outcomes.

Digital measurement in medicine will not replace clinics or clinicians entirely, nor would we want them to. The delivery of, for example, intravenous drugs or surgery, and the value that patients place on their relationship with their provider, cannot be replaced by digital tools. Nonetheless, when used appropriately, digital measurements can improve care by giving clinicians more complete information. Also, transferring some practices out of the clinic and into patients' regular lives – for example, passively measuring sleep quality with wearables instead of requiring overnight stays in clinics – can enhance access to care and reduce cost.

Continuous at-home monitoring also raises a new set of practical issues:

- who will monitor the data?
- who will be responsible for acting on it if it indicates a need for action?
- how will providers be compensated for these tasks?

Although organizations like the Clinical Trials Transformation Initiative (CTTI) have made inroads in addressing the first two questions, the field will need to address these issues and adopt consensus solutions for these tools to be truly integrated into clinical care.[2]

A defining moment for any medical product, whether drug or device, is when the product goes to market. From this perspective, the industry splits into 'premarket' research activities, drug and device development in the life sciences and biotech, and 'postmarket' commercial activities, where the products are used in clinical applications like in the hospital. Often, government regulators like the US Food and Drug Administration (FDA) or the Office for Human Research Protections (OHRP) are the gatekeepers between what is considered research (premarket) and what is part of standard of care and commercial activities (postmarket).

National governments are responsible for establishing national medicines and medical device standards and regulatory authorities that determine what claims product manufacturers can make when they go to market in that country.[3] As of 2015, 121 of the 194 members of the World Health Organization had a national regulatory authority responsible for implementing and enforcing product regulations specific to medical devices.[4] For example, in the USA, the FDA serves this function. Across the Atlantic, this oversight is provided by the European Medicines Agency (EMA) and in Japan, the Pharmaceuticals and Medical Device Agency (PMDA).

Key points – where does digital medicine fit?

- Digital medicine holds the promise of bringing complex medical measurements, observations and interventions outside the clinic.
- Clinical research uses include interventional and non-interventional trials, although many practicalities and data management issues are yet to become commodities.
- Regulation of digital medicine varies widely across the globe.

References

1. Department of Health and Human Services. Definitions (CFR 46.102). In: *Part 46 Protection of Human Subjects; Subpart A – Basic HHS Policy for Protection of Human Research*, 2009. www.hhs.gov/ohrp/sites/default/files/ohrp/policy/ohrpregulations.pdf, last accessed 31 July 2019.

2. Clinical Trials Transformation Initiative. *Recommendations Executive Summary: Advancing the Use of Mobile Technologies for Data Capture & Improved Clinical Trials*, 2018. www.ctti-clinicaltrials.org/sites/www.ctti-clinicaltrials.org/files/mobile-technologies-executive-summary.pdf, last accessed 31 July 2019.

3. World Health Organization. *Medicines Regulatory Support*. www.who.int/medicines/areas/quality_safety/regulation_legislation/en/, last accessed 31 July 2019.

4. World Health Organization. *Global Atlas of Medical Devices*. Geneva: World Health Organization, 2017. www.who.int/medical_devices/publications/global_atlas_meddev2017/en/, last accessed 31 July 2019.

3 Regulatory considerations

There are countless articles and books that discuss regulatory considerations associated with medical product development. We will keep this chapter brief and provide key concepts and frameworks to consider.

It is essential to understand that regulatory agencies like the US Food and Drug Administration (FDA) regulate medical products (like drugs and diagnostic devices) but not the practice of medical care. Structurally, the FDA has six centers, with three most relevant to digital medicine developers:

- Center for Drug Evaluation and Research (CDER)
- Center for Biologics Evaluation and Research (CBER)
- Center for Devices and Radiological Health (CDRH).[1]

Drugs and biologics

Clinical trials for drug and biologic development are organized across phases (Figure 3.1), and the results of these trials are reported to the CDER or CBER, respectively.

Preclinical studies test the drug in vitro (test tube or cell culture) and in vivo (animal models).

Phase 0 started as an informal stage designation that companies used to describe non-drug studies that are exploratory to prepare for the upcoming or ongoing drug research. During this phase, methods of measurement or specialized techniques may be tested without the risks associated with administering an investigational medicine. In 2006, this phase was formalized by FDA guidance to include studies that use tiny doses of a drug (< 1% of expected therapeutic dose) in healthy volunteers to determine if the chemical properties of the drug warrant further development.[2]

Phase I 'first in human' trials test the drugs in healthy human participants. The goal of this phase is to assess the safety and

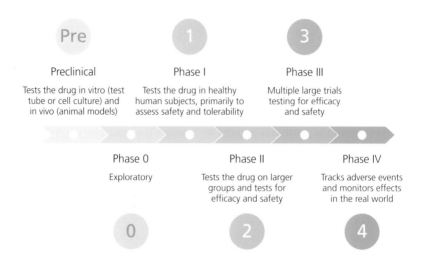

Figure 3.1 The phases of clinical trial research. Clinical trials pass through a series of phases as the trial sponsor gains more evidence around the investigational drug or biologic. Preclinical studies are often conducted in cell and animal models (e.g. on mice) and then are slowly expanded into humans: first in healthy humans in small numbers to test safety, and then to larger sets of humans who have the condition in question to test both safety and efficacy.

tolerability of the drug by starting with low doses on a small number of healthy people (e.g. < 15 participants) and progressively increasing the doses toward the expected effective concentration. Safety is monitored and measured in all subsequent phases as well. These studies are often conducted in highly controlled and specialized inpatient clinics.

Phase II trials enroll larger groups of patients with the medical condition of interest and begin to test for efficacy, while attempting to establish dose and frequency schedules for the final drug product.

Phase III is most often the 'pivotal' stage of testing in which definitive evidence of efficacy and safety must be developed in multiple large trials. The endpoints of these trials ultimately serve as the evidence for the label claims that regulatory agencies allow pharmaceutical companies to use when marketing a drug.

Phase IV trials, also known as observational or postmarketing surveillance, are a hybrid of research and clinical care. In these trials, the drug is already licensed for use and is being prescribed to patients. The purpose of Phase IV trials is to monitor the effects of these new therapies to identify and evaluate previously unreported adverse reactions. Phase IV trials allow sponsors (biopharma and device manufacturers) to see how the product is performing in the 'real world'. These trials also provide an opportunity to test the therapy in new demographics and find new markets, often resulting in label expansion, where the sponsor can make claims that the drug works for additional types of patients/diseases beyond the original use (Box 3.1).

BOX 3.1

Real-world data

Clinical trials in all phases are increasingly including data captured during routine clinical care, such as electronic healthcare records and claims data. This is driven in large part by the passage of the 21st Century Cures Act, which tasked the FDA with considering this type of data during the approval of new medical products.

Novel digital tools

Novel digital tools are being adopted at different rates in different stages of clinical trials, most likely because different trial stages are associated with different levels of risk to the sponsor. Phase III is an unlikely place to see novel measurements of any kind, as disrupting a large complex trial and risking the primary endpoint(s) could be expensive and harmful to the development process. In contrast, implementing exploratory efficacy measures in a small early-stage safety trial may be inexpensive and introduce minimal risk to the primary endpoint(s). Sponsors are now deploying digital tools in Phase I, II and III trials as digital measurements need to be relatively consistent in the early stages of trials to develop the necessary evidence both for internal decision-making and regulatory approval.

The regulatory terms that describe tools, methods, materials or measures that can potentially facilitate the medical product's development are drug development tools (DDTs) or medical device development tools (MDDTs) ('tools' are different from 'devices' at the FDA).[3,4] The FDA has also released a request for comments on prescription drug-use-related software (PDURS) for software that is developed for use with prescription drugs (including biological drug products), which may include, but is not limited to, tracking drug ingestion, calculating the appropriate dose, sending reminders to take the drug or providing information on how to use a drug.[5]

There are also combination products, which contain both a drug and software that meets the definition of a device because of its function.[6] For example, Abilify MyCite is a drug-device combination product comprised of aripiprazole tablets embedded with a software-based ingestible event marker intended to track drug ingestion. Patients can opt to share these data with their healthcare providers or caregivers.[5]

Medical devices

Similar to the approval process in the FDA's CDER and CBER, medical devices in the CDRH go through a process for clearance or approval. However, because medical devices have more predictable effects than a novel chemical might have when introduced into the body, regulators generally pay more attention to technical and design aspects of the product when considering safety. This is particularly true for those devices that operate non-invasively, and thus are less risky. All novel drugs are considered dangerous until proven otherwise, but medical device studies can be adjudicated as posing a non-significant risk based on design criteria.[7]

The CDRH is often the point of contact for digital medicine developers who are building digital medical products such as 'software as a medical device' (SaMD).[8] A 'device' is a term of art at the FDA, which means that it has a precise and specialized meaning. The CDRH is responsible for regulating digital 'devices' but not digital tools. As such, we limit our use of the term 'device' in this book to be consistent with the FDA's definition for a 'medical device' (see FDA 2013 and 2017).[9,10]

For the US market, it is important to distinguish that the FDA does not regulate what the product actually does, but rather what an organization claims the product does. For instance, let us say Product A and Product B are exactly the same mobile sensor technology, i.e. the same hardware, firmware and software/algorithm that produce a measurement. If Product A states that the intended use of this measurement is for a wellness purpose, it likely is not regulated. If Product B says the intended use of this measurement is to make a diagnosis, then it would be considered a 'device' and regulated by the FDA. This means that the exact same product can be developed and marketed either as a 'device' (and thus, regulated) or not a device (and unregulated) simply through a change of words, and no change in hardware or code.

At the time of this publication, for example, a Fitbit is not regulated by the FDA as it does not claim to serve a medical purpose. Therefore, a Fitbit is considered a digital measurement tool or a mobile sensor technology but not a 'device'.

Put another way: asking 'is my digital product a medical device?' is not the most useful question. A better question would be about the intended use of the product (i.e. is the organization making a medical device claim?). Generally, answering this question is not easy, which is why many software manufacturers will spend millions of dollars on regulatory consultants. The FDA has an open-door policy and encourages organizations to come early and often during product development. It is good practice to initiate the conversation about regulatory designation of the product early. A good starting point is with the FDA's Division of Industry and Consumer Education (DICE).[11]

As tools develop multiple functions (e.g. can measure step count, heart rate and tremor and can be tailored to specific populations), these digital measurement technologies may be used for either medical product development or commercial clinical care activities.[12] Whether the software is a 'device' is ultimately determined by a regulatory body and likely will depend upon the software's intended functions.

Medical devices can presumptively be classified by risk profile, currently defined by the FDA as Class I, II or III in order of increasing risk.

Class I devices require little safety testing. Today, around 50% of medical devices fall under this category and 95% of these are exempt from the regulatory process.[13,14]

Class II devices. Of note, many medical device companies, including digital medicine developers, will bypass Class I and strive to get their devices categorized as at least Class II, because this category is generally the lowest risk class that is also covered by insurance, enabling greater access. Notably, Apple's first FDA-cleared product, an electrocardiogram (EKG) over-the-counter (e.g. non-prescription) app, was categorized as Class II.[15]

Class III devices pose a high risk to the patient and/or user (e.g. they sustain or support life, are implanted or present potential unreasonable risk of illness or injury). These types of devices represent around 10% of devices regulated by the CDRH.[14] Implantable pacemakers and breast implants are examples of Class III devices.

Regulatory pathways. Devices that perform a similar function to an existing device on the market (a predicate) can be approved simply by demonstrating that they are at least as effective and no more dangerous than the existing device. This pathway is called 510(k) clearance. As devices increase in risk – meaning they have the potential to cause harm either by malfunctioning or by providing bad information – there becomes more of a burden on the manufacturer to demonstrate safety and efficacy, both from a technical perspective and in controlled human trials.

Historically, the focus of the CDRH relied heavily on the concept of a 'predicate', a legally marketed device (e.g. already on the market) with which a new device would claim equivalence. Whether or not a proposed device has a predicate impacts the regulatory pathway the device can use. For instance, a 'de novo' classification does not require comparison with an existing device on the market.

Notably, in the fall of 2018, the FDA made a sweeping announcement that it is planning an overhaul to de-emphasize its predicate process. While this is probably a positive move to better treat patients, it will take some years to move away from the current system.[16]

FDA-approved versus FDA-cleared. Many people do not realize that there is a difference.

- 'Approved' indicates that the device successfully completed an FDA premarket approval (PMA), which evaluates the safety and effectiveness of Class III high-risk products.
- 'Cleared' indicates that the device successfully completed a 510(k) pathway (see page 32), which is for lower-risk-level products (Table 3.1). Technically, de novos are 'granted', though colloquially people will often say 'cleared' to indicate either the 510(k) or de novo process.

For those looking to learn more about US regulatory considerations for digital products, it is a Herculean task to comb through existing FDA 'guidances with digital health content'.[17] A good starting point includes the guidance on General Wellness: Policy for Low Risk Devices, Mobile Medical Applications, SaMD and Clinical and Patient

TABLE 3.1

Regulatory pathways for device development

Regulatory pathway	510(k)	De novo	Premarket approval
Product risk levels	Class I and II	Class I and II	Class III
FDA decision type	Cleared	Granted	Approved
Requires a predicate	Yes	No	No
Decision criteria	Product demonstrates 'substantial equivalence' to a predicate (e.g. no independent assessment of the product required)	Probable benefits of the product outweigh probable risks	Requires independent assessment of the product's safety and effectiveness

Decision Support (CDS and PDS, respectively) Software.[18-21] The FDA has been taking a forward-looking stance on how to handle digital products, including machine learning and algorithms, and streamline the regulatory process.

Software Precertification (Pre-Cert) Program. The FDA is, for example, piloting a Software Precertification (Pre-Cert) Program, with companies like Apple, Fitbit and Samsung participating.[22] This pilot program allows software manufacturers to have a more streamlined review process, which would make it easier to release new software versions to market if the organization is 'precertified'. The Pre-Cert Program draws heavily on the International Medical Device Regulators Forum (IMDRF) definitions and categories for SaMD.[23] SaMDs (e.g. software-only products like apps and algorithms decoupled from a hardware component) may be subject to more flexible regulations than software-in-a-medical device (SiMD; e.g. traditional software contained within a pacemaker).

Defining 'device'. The 21st Century Cures Act (Cures Act), signed into law on 13 December 2016, amended the definition of 'device' in the Food, Drug, and Cosmetic Act to exclude certain software functions, including some described in many existing guidance documents. The FDA has been assessing how to revise its guidance to represent current thinking on this topic. There has been a recent trend to allow more digital products to go straight to market. For instance, the Cures Act made clearer distinctions on what is considered a regulated medical device versus a wellness product or a digital technology that is not a 'device' (e.g. an electronic health record [EHR]).[24] The distinction between those digital products/technologies that are considered medical devices, and those that are not, is a hazy one.

Determining the nature of a digital product is especially challenging because the FDA has other mechanisms like *enforcement discretion*, where the FDA may determine that the product is a 'device', but chooses not to regulate it.[25] As these decisions are continuously evolving, some helpful resources to navigate the area include the Federal Trade Commission's Mobile Health Apps Interactive Tool and DICE.[11,26] There are also papers that draw a comparison of

European and US approval processes (e.g. mapping the European Union [EU] Conformité Européenne [CE] mark to the FDA framework).[27]

In Europe, a working group commissioned by NHS England has developed an 'Evidence Standards Framework for Digital Health Technologies' to make it easier for innovators and regulators to define what 'good' looks like within digital medicine.[28] There are many groups across the world working toward a more streamlined vision. The Digital Medicine Society (DiMe) is developing a resource on its website (www.dimesociety.org) to keep track of the different standards, papers and frameworks.[29]

Decisions that influence classification. Although regulatory authorities have the final say as to whether the digital product is a medical 'device', the organization that develops and markets the product can make many choices that influence the likelihood of it being classified as a medical device. For example, organizations choose what claims to make about the product, how much evidence to gather to support those claims and which markets to enter (and subsequently, which regulatory bodies to be regulated by).

The downstream consequences of these decisions include who can access the product, under what circumstances and for what reasons, and who is likely to pay for such access. Talking with the appropriate regulatory authority early and often is important during the product development process; it will minimize surprises and develop a forward-thinking regulatory strategy.

Put simply, the CDRH is primarily concerned with whether a medical product, including both hardware and software, is safe to use and accurate for measuring what it claims to measure. If the manufacturer of that system does not claim it has a medical use (e.g. diagnostic, monitoring), the product will not be regulated by the CDRH. Agencies that evaluate new drugs and biologics, like the CDER and CBER, care about whether the observation being made by a digital tool (concept of interest) is valid for the way it is being used in regulated research (context of use): for example, if the digital tool is being used to measure an endpoint in the clinical trial.

Table 3.2 is a 'cheat sheet' of the primary pathways to market through the CDRH for a software product.

TABLE 3.2

'If my software product is regulated by the FDA, how do I bring it to market?'

Go-to-market strategy	Risk classification options	Is product making a 'device' claim?[a]	Can manufacturer bring the product straight to market?	Does manufacturer need to 'register and list'?
• Not a device • Not regulated by FDA	N/A, not a device	No	Yes	No
• Is a device • FDA will exercise 'enforcement discretion' and will not regulate it	Class I or II	Yes	Yes	No
• Is a device • Is exempt from review by the FDA	Class I or II	Yes	Yes	Yes
• Is a device • Will be reviewed under the FDA Pre-Cert program	Class I, II or III[f]	Yes	No	Yes
• Is a device • Will be reviewed under a traditional CDRH pathway (e.g. 510[k], de novo or PMA)	Class I, II or III	Yes	No	Yes

[a]For example, what's the intended use?
[b]For example, medical device reporting.
[c]www.ftc.gov/tips-advice/business-center/guidance/mobile-health-apps-interactive-tool
[d]www.fda.gov/medicaldevices/digitalhealth/mobilemedicalapplications/ucm368744.htm
[e]www.fda.gov/medicaldevices/deviceregulationandguidance/overview/classifyyourdevice/ucm051549.htm
[f]Or will fall under the risk determination newly proposed by the International Medical Device Regulators Forum (IMDRF).

Does FDA review the product?	Is manufacturer required to submit postmarket information?[b]	Does manufacturer need to pass a pre-cert excellence appraisal?	Is pathway 'live'?	Related documents (see footnotes)
No	No	No	Yes	Mobile health apps interactive tool (HHS, ONC, OCR and FDA)[c]
No	No	No	Yes	Examples of mobile apps for which the FDA will exercise enforcement discretion[d]
No	Yes	No	Yes	Class I/II exemptions[e]
Yes	Yes	Yes	Yes	Digital Health Software Precertification (Pre-Cert) Program[g]
Yes	Yes	No	Yes	FDA DICE[h]

[g]www.fda.gov/MedicalDevices/DigitalHealth/DigitalHealthPreCertProgram/default.htm
[h]www.fda.gov/medicaldevices/deviceregulationandguidance/
contactdivisionofindustryandconsumereducation/default.htm
CDRH: Center for Devices and Radiological Health; DICE, Division of Industry and Consumer Education; FDA, US Food and Drug Administration; HHS, Health and Human Services; OCR, Office for Civil Rights; ONC, Office of the National Coordinator for Health Information Technology; PMA, premarket approval.

Key points – regulatory considerations

- Agencies such as the US Food and Drug Administration (FDA) regulate what manufacturers claim a product can do (rather than what a product actually does), which means that a product can be considered a 'device' (and regulated) or not a device (and not regulated) through only a change in words and no change to hardware or software.
- Digital measurement tools that are considered a 'device' are regulated by the FDA Center for Devices and Radiological Health (CDRH). Digital tools that support drug applications (e.g. those that capture digital endpoint data) are regulated by the FDA Center for Drug Evaluation and Research (CDER).
- Increasingly more manufacturers of digital products are considering the 'de novo' regulatory pathway so they do not have to deal with predicates and can develop an application that better reflects the software's unique characteristics.
- The regulatory frameworks for digital tools are in flux, and developers should continue to read upcoming guidance, comment on the revisions in the public docket and engage in the process to improve regulatory decision-making.

References

1. US Food and Drug Administration. *History of FDA's Centers and Offices,* 2018. www.fda.gov/about-fda/ history-fdas-internal-organization/ history-fdas-centers-and-offices, last accessed 31 July 2019.

2. Fromer MJ. FDA introduces new phase 0 for clinical trials: some enthusiastic, some skeptical. *Oncol Times* 2006;28:18–19.

3. US Food and Drug Administration. *Drug Development Tool Qualification Programs,* 2019. www.fda.gov/drugs/ development-approval-process-drugs/ drug-development-tool-qualification-programs, last accessed 31 July 2019.

4. US Food and Drug Administration. *Medical Device Development Tools (MDDT),* 2019. www.fda.gov/medical-devices/science-and-research-medical-devices/medical-device-development-tools-mddt, last accessed 31 July 2019.

5. US Food and Drug Administration. Prescription drug use related software; Establishment of public docket. Request for comments. *Federal Register* 2018;83(244): 58574–82. www.federalregister.gov/ documents/2018/11/20/2018-25206/ prescription-drug-use-related-software-establishment-of-a-public-docket-request-for-comments, last accessed 31 July 2019.

6. US Food and Drug Administration. *Combination Products.* Available from: www.fda.gov/combination-products, last accessed 31 July 2019.

7. US Food and Drug Administration. *Significant Risk and Nonsignificant Risk Medical Device Studies,* 2006. www.fda.gov/downloads/ RegulatoryInformation/Guidances/ UCM126418.pdf, last accessed 31 July 2019.

8. US Food and Drug Administration. *Software as a Medical Device (SaMD),* 2018. www.fda.gov/medical-devices/ digital-health/software-medical-device-samd, last accessed 31 July 2019.

9. US Food and Drug Administration. *Is The Product a Medical Device?* 2018. www.fda.gov/medical-devices/ classify-your-medical-device/ product-medical-device, last accessed 31 July 2019.

10. US Food and Drug Administration. *Changes to Existing Medical Software Policies Resulting from Section 3060 of the 21st Century Cures Act,* 2017. www.fda.gov/regulatory-information/search-fda-guidance-documents/changes-existing-medical-software-policies-resulting-section-3060-21st-century-cures-act, last accessed 31 July 2019.

11. US Food and Drug Administration. *Contact Us – Division of Industry and Consumer Education (DICE).* www.fda.gov/medical-devices/device-advice-comprehensive-regulatory-assistance/ contact-us-division-industry-and-consumer-education-dice, last accessed 31 July 2019.

12. US Food and Drug Administration. *Multiple Function Device Products: Policy and Considerations*, 2018. www.fda.gov/ regulatory-information/search-fda-guidance-documents/multiple-function-device-products-policy-and-considerations, last accessed 31 July 2019.

13. US Food and Drug Administration. *Reclassification*, 2018. www.fda.gov/medical-devices/ classify-your-medical-device/ reclassification, last accessed 31 July 2019.

14. BMP Medical. *What's the Difference Between the FDA Medical Device Classes?* 2018. www. bmpmedical.com/blog/whats-difference-fda-medical-device-classes-2/, last accessed 31 July 2019.

15. US Food and Drug Administration. *Device Classification under Section 513(f)(2)(de novo)*. www.accessdata.fda.gov/scripts/ cdrh/cfdocs/cfpmn/denovo. cfm?ID=DEN180044, last accessed 31 July 2019.

16. Burton TM. FDA is revamping clearance procedures for medical devices. *Wall Street Journal* 2018. www.wsj.com/articles/fda-is-revamping-clearance-procedures-for-medical-devices-1543234015, last accessed 31 July 2019.

17. US Food and Drug Administration. Guidances with Digital Health Content, 2018. www.fda.gov/medical-devices/ digital-health/guidances-digital-health-content, last accessed 31 July 2019.

18. US Food and Drug Administration. *General Wellness: Policy for Low Risk Devices*, 2016. www.fda.gov/regulatory-information/ search-fda-guidance-documents/ general-wellness-policy-low-risk-devices, last accessed 31 July 2019.

19. US Food and Drug Administration. *Mobile Medical Applications*, 2015. www.fda.gov/ downloads/MedicalDevices/ DeviceRegulationandGuidance/ GuidanceDocuments/UCM263366. pdf, last accessed 24 September 2019.

20. US Food and Drug Administration. *Software as a Medical Device (SAMD): Clinical Evaluation*, 2017. www.fda.gov/media/100714/ download, last accessed 31 July 2019.

21. US Food and Drug Administration. *Clinical and Patient Decision Software*, 2017. www.fda.gov/ regulatory-information/search-fda-guidance-documents/clinical-and-patient-decision-support-software, last accessed 31 July 2019.

22. US Food and Drug Administration. *Digital Health Software Precertification (Pre-Cert) Program*, 2019. www.fda.gov/ medical-devices/digital-health/ digital-health-software-precertification-pre-cert-program, last accessed 31 July 2019.

23. International Medical Device Regulators Forum. *Software as a Medical Device (SaMD)* [work complete – historical reference]. www.imdrf.org/workitems/wi-samd. asp, last accessed 31 July 2019.

24. US Food and Drug Administration. *21st Century Cures Act*, 2018. www.fda.gov/regulatory-information/selected-amendments-fdc-act/21st-century-cures-act, last accessed 31 July 2019.

25. US Food and Drug Administration. *Examples of Mobile Apps for Which the FDA Will Exercise Enforcement Discretion*, 2018. www.fda.gov/medical-devices/mobile-medical-applications/examples-mobile-apps-which-fda-will-exercise-enforcement-discretion, last accessed 31 July 2019.

26. Federal Trade Commission. *Mobile Health Apps Interactive Tool*, 2016. www.ftc.gov/tips-advice/business-center/guidance/mobile-health-apps-interactive-tool, last accessed 31 July 2019.

27. Van Norman GA. Drugs and devices: comparison of European and US approval processes. *JACC Basic Transl Sci* 2016; 1:399–412.

28. National Institute for Health and Care Excellence. *Evidence Standards Framework for Digital Health Technologies*, 2019. www.nice.org.uk/Media/Default/About/what-we-do/our-programmes/evidence-standards-framework/digital-evidence-standards-framework.pdf, last accessed 31 July 2019.

29. The Digital Medicine Society. The Digital Medicine (DiMe) Society, 2019. www.dimesociety.org, last accessed 30 July 2019.

4 Ethical principles and our responsibilities

As more digital tools are deployed in health research and care settings, new questions emerge about how to use them responsibly and ethically. Anyone developing and/or testing a digital tool for use in disease prevention and treatment within the USA should be aware of the regulatory requirement to obtain institutional review board (IRB) approval prospectively when involving people as research participants.

History

The development of the IRB peer review process stemmed from egregious acts whereby researchers disregarded the rights and welfare of research participants. One example, known as the 'Tuskegee Study of Untreated Syphilis in the Negro Male', was an observational study of the natural progression of syphilis initiated by the Public Health Services in 1932.[1,2] At that time, there was no treatment for syphilis; however, after penicillin was developed, the study participants were not treated and the study continued for nearly 40 years. The National Research Act was passed in 1974; it involved creating a National Commission for the Protection of Human Subjects of Biomedical and Behavioral Research with a goal of preventing future atrocities. It was this Commission that required the formation of IRBs and also wrote the Belmont Report. Published in 1979, the Belmont Report describes three guiding principles of ethical biomedical and behavioral research: respect for persons, beneficence and justice.

As cybersecurity concerns increased with research involving information and communication technologies (ICT), the Department of Homeland Security developed the Menlo Report. Published in 2012, this Report adapted the ethical principles of the Belmont Report to ICT research and added a fourth principle – that of respect for the law and public interest, which focuses on transparence of potential conflicting interests and accountability of stakeholders.[3]

Informed by guiding ethical principles, a federal policy for the protection of human subjects was published in 1991 and adopted by 15 federal agencies and institutes.[4] The regulations speak to basic protections for human research participants in subpart A, known as the Common Rule. Additional subparts speak to protections for vulnerable populations, including children and prisoners.

Core principles

Here, we describe the ethical principles and how the regulations and Common Rule are implemented in practice. The three core principles of biomedical ethics described in the Belmont Report are at the core of research ethics and should be carefully considered during the study design phase and ethics review process.[5]

Respect for persons is demonstrated through the informed consent process, which occurs when a person is given the information needed to make a sound decision about whether to volunteer to willingly participate. How this information is conveyed is important because volunteering to be a research participant is different from, say, accepting terms of service (ToS) to access an app, or signing a consent form to obtain medical care. In the latter, a person will not be able to access the app if they do not accept the ToS nor will they receive medical care if they do not sign the medical consent form. Consent to participate in research is a choice that an individual can only make if presented with information in a setting conducive to good decision-making. There can be no coercive actions (e.g. high incentive payments, free services) that may compromise an individual's ability to volunteer. The informed consent process involves more than signing a form to document voluntary participation – it is the first of what may be many interactions between a participant and the research team and is part of developing a trusted relationship.

Technological literacy is another important consideration. For informed consent to be meaningful, participants will need to be 'tech-literate' enough to understand the specifics of how their data will be obtained and used. Likewise, concerns about privacy are often raised when discussing the passive and ubiquitous nature of the tools used in digital medicine.[6] Attitudes and preferences also vary across generations, with older adults preferring more privacy control compared with teens and young adults.[7]

Education. All these concerns suggest a need to better educate prospective participants – and yet, integrating these concepts into the consent process is not easy. Moving forward, this charge will require a commitment from the medical community to provide accessible public-facing educational modules. For example, one way to improve tech literacy might be to include a brief animation describing the difference between de-identification and anonymity when describing data-sharing practices, or an illustration of what it means to store data in a cloud. A participant may also think that if the study team has access to their health data in real time, 24/7, then that means someone is paying attention to them (which may not be the case). Clarifying these concepts is important and how best to do this will require experts in instructional design who can deliver creative educational content. One organization working to advance meaningful informed consent in digital health research is Sage Bionetworks; it has published a toolkit to assist researchers.[8]

Beneficence is where the probability and magnitude of potential harms are weighed against the possible benefits to a participant, the people they represent and society. Determining risk of harm is a somewhat subjective process, yet worth breaking down. We need to consider potential sources of harm and try to quantify the likelihood of something going wrong as well as the consequences. For instance, if a technology collects and then transmits a study participant's location data to a publicly accessible or non-secure website, the likelihood of a loss of privacy is 100% for all users – yet the consequences will vary. For most people, these will be negligible, but for a domestic abuse survivor or undocumented migrant, the consequences might be severe. Thus, the same potential harm presents a low risk for most, but a high risk for some important groups.

Safeguarding data and managing data-sharing protocols are important considerations when applying the principle of beneficence, and researchers, IRBs and research participants need to think about carefully these. When using third-party commercial apps or measurement tools, it is critical that ToS and end user license agreements (EULAs) be reviewed to ensure they do not introduce unnecessary risks to the end user, be it a research participant or patient.

Harm. Other factors specific to risk assessment include the type of potential harm (e.g. physical, psychological, economic, social) as well as the duration and severity of harm to research participants. Research is inherently risky because we are learning something that is not yet known. Research participants are often told about risks as an odds ratio. For example, in studies that include a test for maximum oxygen uptake, participants are required to exercise to exhaustion. There is a 1 in 12000 chance that a healthy individual doing this study will have a cardiac event that may lead to death. Because of this particular risk of harm, the research team can mitigate risk by having access to personnel and equipment used to treat a cardiac event. Having this information, an individual can decide whether they want to take that chance or not.

Validity and reliability. Within the domain of beneficence is the need for the digital measurement tools to be valid and reliable (see chapter 9). There is no potential benefit of knowledge gain if the study is poorly designed and the tools are not trustworthy. The old adage 'garbage in, garbage out' is a serious concern and one that must be addressed by doing the appropriate studies early to ensure the products, regardless of whether there is a medical claim, are safe and produce useful data.

Justice. The principle of justice focuses on the fair distribution of the benefits and burdens of research and recruitment protocols that are inclusive of those most likely to benefit from knowledge gained. With digital tools, we have the opportunity to reach a more diverse audience, including those in communities where health disparities are most prevalent. To do that requires that we design technologies that are accessible and, in some cases, culturally tailored. With that in mind, including end users in the development process who represent a wide cross-section of our society is one way we can be responsive to the principle of justice.

For example, in a study designed to increase physical activity in refugee women, the researcher decided to use a wrist-worn accelerometer to assess daily movement. The participants were given the sensor and shown how to use it. One week later, the researcher returned to gather the measurement tools and found that no data had been collected. Turns out a wrist-worn mobile technology was culturally unacceptable and drew unwanted attention to the women, so they did not wear it.[9] This story sheds light on the fact that while digital tools should improve access to health research and healthcare, they can also perpetuate disparities and prevent access if not well designed and deployed.

Key points – ethical principles and our responsibilities

- The principles that guide the ethical conduct of biomedical and behavioral research include: respect for persons, beneficence, justice (Belmont Report) and respect for law and public interest (Menlo Report).
- Knowing how to apply ethical principles is a responsibility of all stakeholders involved in digital health research, including technologists, researchers and ethics review boards.

References

1. Centers for Disease Control and Prevention. *US Public Health Service Syphilis Study at Tuskegee. The Tuskegee Timeline*, 2016. www.cdc.gov/tuskegee/timeline.htm, last accessed 25 August 2019.

2. Chadwick GL. Historical perspective: Nuremberg, Tuskegee, and the radiation experiments. *J Int Assoc Physicians AIDS Care* 1997;3:27–8.

3. US Department of Homeland Security. *The Menlo Report: Ethical Principles Guiding Information and Communication Technology Research*, 2012. www.dhs.gov/sites/default/files/publications/CSDMenloPrinciplesCORE-20120803_1.pdf, last accessed 24 September 2019.

4. Office for Human Research Protections. *Federal Policy for the Protection of Human Subjects ('Common Rule')*, 2016. www.hhs.gov/ohrp/regulations-and-policy/regulations/common-rule/index.html, last accessed 24 September 2019.

5. The National Commission for the Protection of Human Subjects of Biomedical and Behavioral Research, Department of Health, Education and Welfare (DHEW). *The Belmont Report*. Washington: US Government Printing Office, 1978. https://videocast.nih.gov/pdf/ohrp_belmont_report.pdf, last accessed 31 July 2019.

6. Filkins BL, Kim JY, Roberts B et al. Privacy and security in the era of digital health: what should translational researchers know and do about it? *Am J Transl Res* 2016;8:1560–80.

7. Wang S, Bolling K, Mao W et al. Technology to support aging in place: the older adult perspective. *Healthcare* 2019;7:E60.

8. Sage Bionetworks. *Elements of Informed Consent*, 2019. https://sagebionetworks.org/tools_ resources/elements-of-informed-consent, last accessed 25 August 2019.

9. Nebeker C, Murray K, Holub C et al. Acceptance of mobile health in communities underrepresented in biomedical research: barriers and ethical considerations for scientists. *JMIR Mhealth Uhealth* 2017;5:e87.

5 Ethics in practice

Because of past harms associated with research involving human participants, there is an expectation and, in many cases, a regulatory requirement that an ethics committee review will take place in advance of the research commencing. In research supported by the US Department of Health and Human Services (HHS) or under US Food and Drug Administration (FDA) oversight, this is carried out by an institutional review board (IRB) registered with the federal Office for Human Research Protections (OHRP).[1] These regulations were initiated in 1974 as part of the National Research Act.

The involvement of an IRB in behavioral and biomedical research is common globally, though often by other names, such as a research ethics board (REB) or 'research ethics committee'. An IRB can be a part of the organization conducting the research (i.e. medical center or university) or operate as an independent fee-for-service entity. In the US, an IRB is required to have a minimum of five people, including scientists, non-scientists and someone who is unaffiliated with the organization. This membership convention has been adopted globally for organizations conducting FDA-regulated research under the International Council for Harmonisation of Technical Requirements for Pharmaceuticals for Human Use (ICH) Good Clinical Practice guidelines.[2,3]

The IRB is responsible for reviewing research that involves human participants to evaluate compliance with federal regulations and application of ethical principles. This review includes evaluating the probability and magnitude of potential harms to research participants and weighing these risks against the potential benefits of knowledge to be gained. The IRB also reviews the proposed research to make sure that participants selected to participate represent those most likely to benefit from its results. Moreover, the IRB wants to make sure that people who are invited to participate in research have a good understanding of the study purpose and what they will be asked to do. This process of sharing study information with a prospective participant is called informed consent and is a central tenet of biomedical research.

Federal regulations and accepted ethical principles are in place to guide the conduct of research so that the science is rigorous and the participants are protected. In any research, an important step is to determine if people involved in the testing phase are considered to be human participants in the research. The federal regulations include definitions for what qualifies as 'research' and 'human subject' and address the responsibilities of the organization and research team.[4]

Rather than go into detail here, we suggest that you contact the IRB affiliated with your organization to discuss the process for obtaining approval to test a product on humans. The IRB review and approval are usually needed if the activity is considered to be research and the people involved with testing meet the definition of a human subject (e.g. clinical or non-clinical research). This is true regardless of whether the product is seeking FDA clearance or approval.

IRB review criteria and pathways

Depending on the risk level (e.g. minimal or greater than minimal risk of harm) and type (e.g. psychological, physical, economic), there are three review pathways:
- exempt from the Common Rule
- expedited review
- convened committee.

Exempt from the Common Rule. The exempt classification is appropriate if the study procedures pose no more than a minimal risk of harm (e.g. observation of public activities, survey of adults, analysis of existing data). The concept of minimal risk is defined in the federal regulations and means that the risk to a participant, whether it be physical or psychological, is no greater than what they encounter in normal daily life.[5] When a study is exempt, it means that the Common Rule does not apply to the research. Normally, the IRB decides whether a study meets the criteria for exemption, expedited or full committee review.

Expedited review. To qualify for an expedited review, the study procedures may not exceed minimal risk of harm and must align with one of the criteria described in the regulations.[6] For example, if the research involves collection of biosamples, non-invasive clinical testing (e.g. sensory acuity, moderate exercise by healthy volunteers) or examination of existing data like electronic health records (EHRs), it may be eligible for an expedited review. However, studies that are designed to carry out safety and efficacy testing of a medical device are probably not eligible for an expedited review and will be reviewed by a convened gathering of IRB members. The only difference between an expedited and convened committee review is the number of people involved in evaluating the research plan. An expedited review can be conducted by a subset of the IRB membership, which is usually the IRB chair and one other member.

Convened committee. Any study that does not qualify for exempt or expedited review is evaluated by a convened group of IRB members. For research covered by the Common Rule, documentation of informed consent is required, though this may be waived.

IRB application. Once the type of review is known, an IRB application is developed by the research team that includes a detailed research protocol and a draft of the informed consent document. The protocol will briefly describe the scientific literature that the study is building from, as well as the study aims, procedures, participant inclusion criteria, risks, benefits, risk management, data management, investigator qualifications and informed consent details. The IRB will review this protocol application to evaluate whether the risks are appropriate in relation to the potential contribution to science and benefits to people like those who participate in the study.

Application of ethical principles. Researchers have applied these principles and relied on IRBs to help shape ethical research practices for nearly half a century. However, as digital products are increasingly used in health research and clinical care, all relevant stakeholders have a collective responsibility to think proactively about how to conduct digital health research ethically and responsibly. While IRB approval is an important step in the process for identifying and mitigating risk in studies, it is truly the responsibility of developers, researchers and clinicians to be a part of the ethical decision-making process. Simply stated, we cannot outsource ethics and hope for the best.

Resources

Of course, these regulations and ethical principles are sometimes difficult to put into practice. Because the use of digital methods is relatively new, accessing resources at the protocol development phase is important. Over the past few years, several initiatives have begun to address the ethical, legal and social implications (ELSI) of emerging technologies. A few focus specifically on artificial intelligence (AI) broadly (e.g. autonomous vehicles, facial recognition, city planning, future of work). AI initiatives presently underway (e.g. AI Now, A-100) are well-funded and global collaborative programs. Others addressing digital medicine technologies more specifically include the Connected and Open Research Ethics (CORE) initiative, MobileELSI research project, Sage Bionetworks and the Clinical Trials Transformation Initiative (CTTI), which are described in the following paragraphs.

CORE initiative. Launched in 2015 at the University of California, San Diego, USA, the CORE initiative is a learning 'ethics' resource developed to support the digital medicine research community, including researchers and IRBs. The CORE features a Q&A forum and a resource library with over 100 IRB-approved protocols and consent snippets that have been shared among 700+ members of the CORE Network. All resources are tagged for ease of access. For example, you can search the library to find protocols that have used a digital tool in clinical research involving Latino middle-schoolers or breast cancer survivors (see Figure 5.1).

In addition, the CORE is creating checklists to assist the community in proactive decision-making. One checklist was inspired by a psychiatrist who had recommended to a patient that he use a mobile app to help with managing his daily patterns and mood. On closer inspection of the app's terms of service (ToS) and privacy policy, the clinician realized she was inadvertently putting her patient at

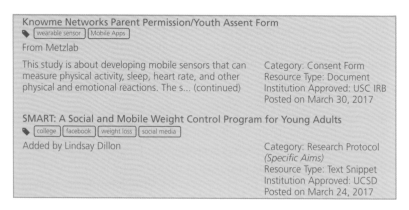

Figure 5.1 Screenshot from the Connected and Open Research Ethics (CORE) Q&A forum.

increased risk because the app was sharing his personal information with third parties. The checklist prompts researchers to think about ethics, privacy, risks and benefits, access and usability, and data management (see http://thecore.ucsd.edu/dmchecklist/) (Figure 5.2).[7]

MobileELSI. The MobileELSI project, led by investigators from Sage Bionetworks and the University of Louisville, has a goal of understanding the scope of unregulated mobile health research to inform the development of a governance model. The increase in public access to technology has led to everyday citizens becoming involved in self-experimentation, a form of 'citizen science', which is largely unregulated as it falls outside of traditional regulatory requirements. In addition, technology companies are increasingly involved in biomedical research. Neither are obligated to apply the federal regulations to protect research participants unless, of course, they are developing an FDA-covered product or are conducting federally funded research. The MobileELSI project will develop recommendations to guide the conduct of unregulated digital medicine research.

Domains • Ethical Principles • Privacy • Risks & Benefits • Access & Usability • Data Management	Ethical principles Place a check to indicate the ethical principle(s) to consider for each item within a domain evaluated			Researcher responsibility	
	Autonomy Actions demonstrate respect for the person	*Beneficence* Actions involve comprehensive risk and benefit assessment	*Justice* Actions demonstrate access to those who may benefit most	Addressed in the research protocol	Addressed during the informed consent process
Privacy (respect for participants)					
Personal information collected is clearly stated				Yes No Unsure	Yes No Unsure
What data are shared is specified				Yes No Unsure	Yes No Unsure
With whom data are shared is stated				Yes No Unsure	Yes No Unsure
Privacy agreement – when a commercial product is used:					
a. Privacy policy is located				Yes No Unsure	Yes No Unsure

Figure 5.2 Excerpt from the Connected and Open Research Ethics (CORE) digital health/medicine decision-making checklist.

Sage Bionetworks and its governance team have led the charge in creating accessible informed consent templates for use on a smartphone that enable digital medicine research. For example, the 'Elements of Informed Consent' toolkit (Figure 5.3) is available to researchers to help them think through developing an effective informed consent process on a mobile device.[8]

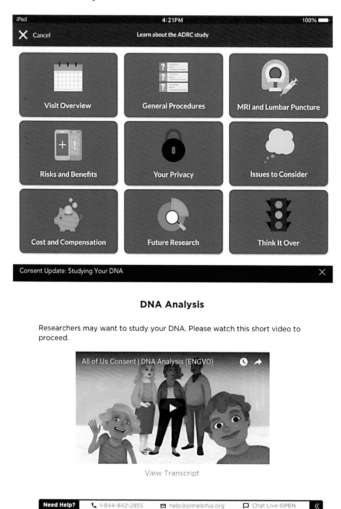

Figure 5.3 Screenshot from Sage Bionetwork's 'Elements of Informed Consent' toolkit.[8]

The CTTI is another source for guidance, with recommendations, resources and practical solutions to support responsible practices in mobile clinical trials.[9]

Ethics when an IRB review is not required

When research involves retrospective analysis of existing data or prospective observation, testing or experimenting with people to generate 'generalizable' knowledge, an IRB review is needed. The term 'generalizable' typically means that the results will be shared through peer-reviewed publication or presentations. The need for IRB review is relatively clear in the world of premarket clinical trials, but the lines defining human research in the postmarket, commercial world have been less obvious.

Some instances of A/B testing may be considered human subject research, depending on whether an organization intends to share knowledge broadly or use it internally to improve its product or service. For example, Facebook found itself in hot water in 2014 after testing different versions of its News Feed with users to study emotional contagion. Had the results been kept internal to Facebook for product improvement, it would have flown under the radar for needing an IRB consult. However, those involved decided to publish the study results to share knowledge produced with the public.

Sharing knowledge is believed by research ethicists and the scientific community to be a responsibility to society – which is certainly a good thing. In this case, though, many users were outraged about being involved in research that they did not consent to. In effect, more than 800 000 Facebook users had become inadvertent research participants.[10,11]

The takeaway message here is that ToS and end user license agreements (EULAs) are not a substitute for informed consent.[12] People want the right to opt-in to being involved in biomedical research, and that is a clear call for respecting the ethical principle of 'respect for persons'. Yet, when we are doing work that is technically not research, what is our ethical obligation? In software development, the way user data have been treated has an emerging history of malfeasance. This practice likely results from the lack of universally agreed guidelines and standards. We strongly recommend the adoption of ethical principles to guide responsible practice when guidelines are lacking.

In response to the lack of guidelines and exploitation of consumer data, new regulations have emerged that speak to consent and privacy concerns. The General Data Protection Regulations (GDPR) were passed by the European Parliament in 2016 and took effect in April 2018. The GDPR were designed to harmonize European Union (EU) privacy laws, protect EU citizens' data privacy and change how organizations, regardless of where they are located, process and manage EU citizen data. An important change that the GDPR introduced was the need for companies to obtain explicit informed consent separate from a ToS or EULA.

This shift from consumers being helpless data subjects to empowered actors in the digital data economy is moving to the US. In 2018, California passed the California Consumer Privacy Act (CCPA) which, when implemented in 2020, gives consumers control over their data and requires that companies like Facebook and Google explain what data they collect, what they do with the data, and who the data are shared with.[13]

Key points – ethics in practice

- Federal regulations and accepted ethical principles are in place to guide the conduct of research so that the science is rigorous and the participants are protected.
- Terms of service and end user license agreements are not a substitute for informed consent.
- Lack of guidelines and exploitation of consumer data have led to new regulations that speak to consent and privacy concerns, including the General Data Protection Regulations in the European Union and the California Consumer Privacy Act.
- Globally, it is common to conduct an ethics review of behavioral and biomedical research; this is carried out by an institutional review board (IRB), a research ethics board or a research ethics committee.
- While IRB approval is an important step in the process for identifying and mitigating risk in studies, it is truly the responsibility of developers, researchers and clinicians to be a part of the ethical decision-making process.
- Because digital measurement methods are relatively new, accessing resources and asking questions at the protocol development phase are critical.

References

1. Bloss C, Nebeker C, Bietz M et al. Reimagining human research protections for 21st century science. *J Med Internet Res* 2016;18:e329.

2. Vijayananthan A, Nawawi O. The importance of Good Clinical Practice guidelines and its role in clinical trials. *Biomed Imaging Interv J* 2008;4:e5.

3. International Council for Harmonisation of Technical Requirements for Pharmaceuticals for Human Use. *Guideline for Good Clinical Practice E6(R2)*. Available from: www.ema.europa.eu/documents/scientific-guideline/ich-e-6-r2-guideline-good-clinical-practice-step-5_en.pdf, last accessed 5 December 2019.

4. Department of Health and Human Services. To what does this policy apply? (CFR 46.101). In: *Part 46 Protection of Human Subjects; Subpart A – Basic HHS Policy for Protection of Human Research Subjects*, 2009. www.hhs.gov/ohrp/sites/default/files/ohrp/policy/ohrpregulations.pdf, last accessed 24 September 2019.

5. Department of Health and Human Services. Definitions for purposes of this policy (CFR 46.102). In: *Part 46 Protection of Human Subjects; Subpart A – Basic HHS Policy for Protection of Human Research Subjects*, 2009. www.hhs.gov/ohrp/sites/default/files/ohrp/policy/ohrpregulations.pdf, last accessed 31 July 2019.

6. Department of Health and Human Services. Expedited review procedures for certain kinds of research involving no more than minimal risk, and for minor changes in approved research (CFR 46.110). In: *Part 46 Protection of Human Subjects; Subpart A – Basic HHS Policy for Protection of Human Research Subjects,* 2009. www.hhs.gov/ohrp/sites/default/files/ohrp/policy/ohrpregulations.pdf, last accessed 31 July 2019.

7. Nebeker C, Bartlett Ellis R, Torous J. Digital health decision-making framework and checklist: designed for researchers. *ReCODE Health*, 2018. https://recode.health/dmchecklist/, last accessed 31 July 2019.

8. Sage Bionetworks. *Elements of Informed Consent*, 2019. https://sagebionetworks.org/tools_ resources/elements-of-informed-consent, last accessed 25 August 2019.

9. Clinical Trials Transformation Initiative. *Project: Mobile Technologies (MCT)*. www.ctti-clinicaltrials.org/projects/mobile-technologies, last accessed 31 July 2019.

10. Paul SM, Mytelka DS, Dunwiddie CT et al. How to improve R&D productivity: the pharmaceutical industry's grand challenge. *Nat Rev Drug Discov* 2010;9:203–14.

11. Meyer R. Everything we know about Facebook's secret mood manipulation experiment. The Atlantic, 2014. www.theatlantic.com/technology/archive/2014/06/everything-we-know-about-facebooks-secret-mood-manipulation-experiment/373648/, last accessed 31 July 2019.

12. Editorial Board. How Silicon Valley puts the 'con' in consent. *New York Times* 2019. www.nytimes.com/2019/02/02/opinion/internet-facebook-google-consent.html, last accessed 31 July 2019.

13. State of California Department of Justice. *California Consumer Privacy Act (CCPA)*, 2018. https://oag.ca.gov/privacy/ccpa, last accessed 31 July 2019.

6 Security, data rights and governance

New digital tools, such as digital biomarkers, can capture an unprecedented amount of information about users, including fine-grained behavioral and physiological states. Many of these tools are non-invasive and collect data passively, which is certainly more convenient but also runs the risk that people do not understand how much of their digital footprint is being collected or shared.[1] Recently granted patents include a shopping cart that monitors your heart rate and Alexa's new ability to apparently diagnose your cough.[2] Data collected from such technologies could be used by a doctor to make a clinical decision or by an insurer to approve or deny a claim.[1] Society needs to decide how to create systems that will deliver real benefits while protecting citizen privacy and safety.[3]

For example, there is a lot of excitement in the healthcare community about using these tools in postmarket monitoring, or surveillance, to track metrics like safety monitoring and efficacy. Although many of these surveillance techniques in healthcare are still in the early stages, security researchers in the tech world are understandably cautious. Put simply: personalized medicine holds great promise for humanity, but it is not possible to have personalized medicine without some amount of 'surveillance' – indeed, they go hand in hand. As de-identification gets more difficult with the vast amount of data generated for an individual, it is critical to understand, for an entity getting access to our data, who, what and when?[4] Health insurers and data brokers have been vacuuming up personal details on individuals, to create predictions on health costs based on race, marital status, whether you pay your bills on time or even buy plus-size clothing.[5] Similar data have been used to create 'health risk scores' for the opioid crisis, determining who gets access to what types of care.[6] Many biases may not come to light until after more rigorous testing; for instance, researchers have found that Fitbits and other wearables may not accurately track heart rates in people of color.[7] The biases in these types of algorithms are starting to become better documented, exacerbating health disparities – and yet our society lacks clear regulatory interventions or punishment for misuse.[8,9]

We have all heard about the 'Internet of Things' (IoT). What is coming next is the 'Internet of Bodies' (IoB) – a network of smart devices that are attached to or inside our bodies, as defined by Professor Andrea Matwyshyn.[10] Most of the digital tools we have discussed fit within the IoB paradigm. Matwyshyn argues that using the human body as a technology platform raises a number of legal and policy questions for which regulators and judges need to prepare.

Our healthcare system has strong protections for how to store and share a patient's biological specimens, such as a blood or genomic sample – but what about our digital specimens? With the increase in biometric surveillance from these tools, data rights and governance – who gets access to what data and when – become critical.[3]

End user license agreements and terms of service, which gain consent one time on sign-up, are not sufficient as a method to actually inform a person about how their health data – in the form of a digital specimen – will be protected.[11] Our society needs better social contracts with tech platforms that have accessible and meaningful informed consent processes baked into the product itself and can be tailored to adapt as user preferences change over time (Figure 6.1).

As the field of digital medicine, and indeed medicine as a whole, advances a process for the creation and promotion of policies, we need standards to ensure that people are protected from known and unknown harms due to myriad computational and human factors, including both failures of knowledge and failures of intent on the part of developers.

Security and compliance

Any organization that works with personally identifiable information, personal health information and direct access to patients is at a high risk for cyber threats. Today, with the rise of connected products, even a few vulnerable lines of code can have a profound impact on human life. Healthcare has seen a proliferation of vulnerabilities, particularly in connected technologies, many of which are life-critical: for example, Johnson & Johnson's insulin pumps, St Jude Medical's implantable cardiac devices, and the WannaCry ransomware attack, which infected 200 000 computers, many of which were part of a critical hospital

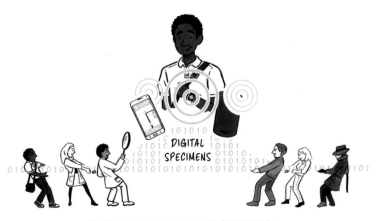

YOUR DIGITAL SPECIMEN IS UP FOR GRABS...
DO YOU KNOW WHO HAS THE RIGHT TO LOOK AT IT?

Figure 6.1 Digital specimens and social contracts. Our healthcare system has strong protections for patients' biological specimens, such as blood samples, but what about our 'digital specimens'? With the increase in biometric surveillance from these tools, data rights and governance – who gets access to what data and when – becomes critical.

infrastructure, across 150 countries.[12-14] Vulnerabilities in connected technologies can be exposed by either black hat or white hat hackers.

- *Black hat* refers to a style of breaking into networks for personal or financial gain, often illegally without the owner's permission.
- *White hat* hackers, also referred to as *security researchers*, perform a style of ethical hacking on mission-critical networks and will employ the policies of coordinated disclosure to the network owner if vulnerabilities are found.[15]

Risk prioritization protocols

A number of organizations have created protocols to prioritize risk levels of known vulnerabilities. For instance, MITRE, a non-profit that operates research and development centers sponsored by the federal government, created the Common Vulnerabilities and Exposures (CVE) program, to identify and catalog vulnerabilities in software or firmware into a free 'dictionary' for organizations to improve their security.[16]

Major agencies that are addressing healthcare cybersecurity include the National Institute of Standards and Technology, which has published a number of well-documented methods for quantitatively and qualitatively assessing cyber risks, and the US Food and Drug Administration (FDA), which has released a number of both premarket and postmarket guidances on cybersecurity best practices.

Implementing protection policies

Researchers and developers should not count on others to implement critical basic protections; they should have knowledge of their organization's policies and important contacts, such as the chief information security officer (CISO). For those embarking on this journey, check out *A cybersecurity primer for translational research*;[17] Box 6.1, for example, comes from this primer and elucidates the concepts of security and compliance, which are often confusing concepts for newcomers to the field.

BOX 6.1

Security and compliance

- Security is the application of protections and management of risk posed by cyber threats.
  - Relates to how the technologies are updated, assessed and used.
- Compliance is typically a top-down mandate based on federal guidelines or law, whereas security is often managed bottom-up and is decentralized in most organizations.
  - Typically relates to documentation (e.g. for the Health Insurance Portability and Accountability Act [HIPAA])

From Perakslis and Stanley, 2016.[17]

Software bill of materials

Most modern software is not written completely from scratch and includes common, off-the-shelf components, modules and libraries from both open-source and commercial teams. A tool to help manage potential vulnerabilities is called a 'software bill of materials' (SBOM), which is analogous to an ingredients list on food packaging and contains all the components in a given piece of software. The FDA has been investing more time and guidance around sharing SBOMs in both pre- and postmarket settings, and so have medical device makers like Philips and Siemens, and healthcare providers like NY Presbyterian and the Mayo Clinic.[18-20]

The Hippocratic Oath for Connected Medical Devices

As monitoring and surveillance tools become mainstream, it is critical to have secure and ethical checks and balances. For example, on graduation from medical school, soon-to-be physicians take the Hippocratic Oath, a symbolic promise to provide care in the best interest of patients. As connected tools increasingly augment clinicians, a critical question emerges: should the manufacturers and adopters of these connected technologies be governed by the symbolic spirit of the Hippocratic Oath?[21]

Inspired by this idea, a number of security researchers from I Am The Cavalry, a grassroots organization with ties to DEF CON, an underground hacking conference, drafted 'The Hippocratic Oath for Connected Medical Devices' (HOCMD).[22] This outlines a number of security and ethical principles, including 'secure by design' and 'resilience and containment'.[21]

While the FDA has not called out the HOCMD by name, in the 3 years since it was published, the FDA has incorporated elements from the five principles across its pre- and postmarket cybersecurity guidelines.[23,24] The FDA has supported further collaboration between security researchers and connected device manufacturers through the agency-led #WeHeartHackers initiative, which launched in early 2019.[25]

In August 2019, over ten medical device manufacturers, including Abbott, Thermo Fischer Scientific, Medtronic, Becton Dickinson, Philips and Siemens, convened at the Biohacking Village at DEF CON with the FDA in attendance. The manufacturers brought over 40 medical devices for white hat hackers to test and attack. The Mayo Clinic set up a model hospital environment where security researchers were able to be in an immersive hospital setting and executed a number of security challenges simulating a real environment. These types of collaborations between regulators, industry and researchers build stronger and more resilient systems for patients and the public health system at large.

Other initiatives

Many government agencies support initiatives to improve security for medical connected technologies and healthcare delivery organizations. For instance, Health and Human Services (HHS) sponsors the Healthcare and Public Health Sector Coordinating Council (HSCC) joint Cybersecurity Working Group (CWG). The mission of the HSCC CWG is to collaborate with HHS and other federal agencies by crafting and promoting the adoption of recommendations and guidance for policy, regulatory and market-driven strategies to facilitate collective mitigation of cybersecurity threats to the sector that affect patient safety, security and privacy and consequently national confidence in the healthcare system.[26]

Key points – security, data rights and governance

- As advances in technology enable digital tools to gather ever larger amounts of high-resolution personal health information, core principles of medical and research ethics must be integrated at every step, beginning in the design phase.
- The line between 'personalization' and 'surveillance' is thin. As a result, and given the near impossibility to 'de-identify' mass amounts of data, it becomes more and more important to know who has access to sensitive data and under what conditions.
- Common practices in the consumer technology industry for obtaining agreement to corporate terms of service, including privacy policies, are not sufficient or appropriate for obtaining informed consent from users, be they patients receiving care or participants in health research. (When was the last time you read an end user license agreement for a website or app you use?)
- The field of digital medicine must develop innovative ways of ensuring that the values of respect, privacy and trust are not lost in the pursuit of better data. It is critical to ensure that the technologies are worthy of the trust we place in them.

References

1. Allen M. You snooze, you lose: insurers make the old adage literally true. *Pro Publica*, 2018. www.propublica.org/article/you-snooze-you-lose-insurers-make-the-old-adage-literally-true, last accessed 31 July 2019.

2. Mehta I. Amazon's new patent will allow Alexa to detect a cough or a cold. *TNW*, 2018. https://thenextweb.com/artificial-intelligence/2018/10/15/amazons-new-patent-will-allow-alexa-to-detect-your-illness/, last accessed 31 July 2019.

3. Perakslis E. Protecting patient privacy and security while exploiting utility of next generation digital heath wearables. *BMJ Opinion*, 2019. https://blogs.bmj.com/bmj/2019/01/18/protecting-patient-privacy-and-security-while-exploiting-the-utility-of-next-generation-digital-health-wearables/, last accessed 31 July 2019.

4. Berinato S. There is no such thing as anonymous data. *Harvard Business Review*, 2015. https://hbr.org/2015/02/theres-no-such-thing-as-anonymous-data, last accessed 31 July 2019.

5. Allen M. Health insurers are vacuuming up details about you—and it could raise your rates. *ProPublica*, 2018. www.propublica.org/article/health-insurers-are-vacuuming-up-details-about-you-and-it-could-raise-your-rates, last accessed 31 July 2019.

6. Ravindranath M. How your health information is sold and turned into risk scores. *Politico*, 2019. www.politico.com/story/2019/02/03/health-risk-scores-opioid-abuse-1139978?mc_cid=e83d0f0d3e&mc_eid=4d57c573ca, last accessed 31 July 2019.

7. Hailu R. Fitbits and other wearables may not accurately track heart rates in people of color. *STAT*, 2019. www.statnews.com/2019/07/24/fitbit-accuracy-dark-skin/, last accessed 24 September 2019.

8. Khullar DA. AI could worsen health disparities. *New York Times*, 2019. www.nytimes.com/2019/01/31/opinion/ai-bias-healthcare.html [paywall], last accessed 31 July 2019.

9. Coravos A, Chen I, Gordhandas A, Stern AD. We should treat algorithms like prescription drugs. *Quartz*, 2019. https://qz.com/1540594/treating-algorithms-like-prescription-drugs-could-reduce-ai-bias/, last accessed 31 July 2019.

10. Matwyshyn AM. The internet of bodies (January 1, 2018). *William & Mary Law Review* 2019;61. Available from SSRN: https://ssrn.com/abstract=3452891.

11. Perakslis E, Coravos A. Is health-care data the new blood? *Lancet Digital Health* 2019;1:PE8–9.

12. Rockoff JD. J&J warns insulin pump vulnerable to cyber hacking. *Wall Street Journal*, 2016. www.wsj.com/articles/j-j-warns-insulin-pump-vulnerable-to-cyber-hacking-1475610989, last accessed 31 July 2019.

13. Larson S. FDA confirms that St. Jude's cardiac devices can be hacked. *CNN Business*, 2017. https://money.cnn.com/2017/01/09/technology/fda-st-jude-cardiac-hack/index.html, last accessed 31 July 2019.

14. Brewster T. Medical devices hit by ransomware for the first time in US hospitals. *Forbes*, 2017. www.forbes.com/sites/thomasbrewster/2017/05/17/wannacry-ransomware-hit-real-medical-devices/#dad2b18425cf, last accessed 31 July 2019.

15. I Am The Cavalry. *I Am The Cavalry Position on Disclosure*, 2018. www.iamthecavalry.org/about/disclosure/, last accessed 31 July 2019.

16. Common Vulnerabilities and Exposures. https://cve.mitre.org, last accessed 31 July 2019.

17. Perakslis ED, Stanley M. A cybersecurity primer for translational research. *Sci Transl Med* 2016;8:322.

18. Philips. *Position Paper: Committed to Proactively Addressing Our Customers Security and Privacy Concerns*, 2018. www.philips.com/cdam/corporate/newscenter/global/standard/resources/healthcare/2018/cybersecurity/Cybersecurity_position_paper.pdf, last accessed 31 July 2019.

19. Aske J, Jacobson J. *NTIA Software Component Transparency: Healthcare Proof of Concept at a Glance*, 2018. www.ntia.doc.gov/files/ntia/publications/healthcare_wg_-_proof_of_concept_overview.pdf, last accessed 31 July 2019.

20. Mayo Clinic. *Medical and Research Device Risk Assessment Vendor Packet Instructions*, 2019. www.mayoclinic.org/documents/medical-device-vendor-instructions/doc-20389647, last accessed 31 July 2019.

21. Woods B, Coravos A, Corman JD. The case for a Hippocratic Oath for Connected Medical Devices: viewpoint. *J Med Internet Res* 2019; 21:e12568.

22. I Am The Cavalry. *Hippocratic Oath for Connected Medical Devices*. www.iamthecavalry.org/domains/medical/oath/, last accessed 31 July 2019.

23. US Food and Drug Administration. *Content of Premarket Submissions for Management of Cybersecurity in Medical Devices*, 2018. www.fda.gov/regulatory-information/search-fda-guidance-documents/content-premarket-submissions-management-cybersecurity-medical-devices, last accessed 31 July 2019.

24. US Food and Drug Administration. *Postmarket Management of Cybersecurity in Medical Devices*, 2016. www.fda.gov/regulatory-information/search-fda-guidance-documents/postmarket-management-cybersecurity-medical-devices, last accessed 31 July 2019.

25. #WeHeartHackers. http://wehearthackers.org, last accessed 31 July 2019.

26. Healthcare and Public Health Sector Critical Infrastructure Security and Resilience Partnership. https://healthsectorcouncil.org, last accessed 31 July 2019.

7 Digital biomarkers and clinical outcomes

Are digital measures the same as digital biomarkers? In some cases, yes. But not always. Determining the best term boils down to what you are measuring and for what purpose. Although we worked hard to minimize jargon in this book, this section will have more technical terms because we strive to use the same language that regulators use to categorize types of measurements, and we want to arm readers with the right language and frameworks to work with regulatory bodies.

The US Food and Drug Administration (FDA) and National Institutes of Health (NIH) came together in 2016 to create the BEST (Biomarkers, EndpointS and other Tools) glossary resource to help clarify terms in this confusing space (Figure 7.1).[1] BEST defines an outcome as any 'measurable characteristic … that is influenced or affected by an individual's baseline state or an intervention as in a clinical trial or other exposure.'

Clinical outcome or biomarker?

The purpose of medicine is to improve health and reduce the risk of an early death. Outcomes are essential measures to determine whether the practice of medicine is working. Outcomes can be clinical outcomes or biomarkers (Box 7.1).

BOX 7.1

Types of measurements in clinical trials

There are multiple types of clinical measurements, including biomarkers, endpoints and outcomes, which are related but take on different meanings in contexts outside of clinical trials.

Biomarker – a defined characteristic that is measured as an indicator of normal biological processes, pathogenic processes, or responses to an exposure or intervention, including therapeutic interventions.

Endpoint – an event or outcome that can be measured objectively to determine whether the intervention being studied is beneficial.

Clinical outcome – describes or reflects how an individual feels, functions or survives.

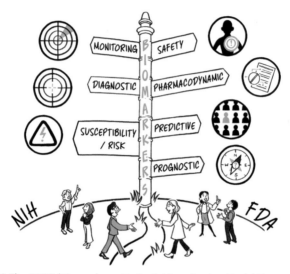

Figure 7.1 The BEST (Biomarkers, EndpointS and other Tools) Framework. In 2016, the US Food and Drug Administration (FDA) and National Institutes of Health (NIH) collaborated to draft 'Biomarkers, EndpointS and other Tools (BEST)', which contains a description of seven types of biomarkers. All of these biomarkers could be measured using digital tools, which results in a digital biomarker.

A clinical outcome 'describes or reflects how an individual feels, functions or survives'.[1] For example, 'average gait speed' for walking bouts greater than a certain number of steps measured over multiple days outside the clinic may be a direct measure of mobility, which is one component of physical functioning.

A biomarker is 'a defined characteristic that is measured as an indicator of normal biological processes, pathogenic processes, or responses to an exposure or intervention, including therapeutic interventions'.[1] For example, a biomarker could be measuring hemoglobin A1c in people with diabetes to determine an individual's average blood sugar level over the past several months.

For biomarkers, think 'signs', not 'symptoms', which are more likely a clinical outcome. Most of the time, biomarker measures are not the things that are necessarily meaningful to patients – but the measurements might be accurate representations, predictors or monitors of underlying biology and disease.

In many circumstances, meaningful clinical outcomes such as survival or the occurrence of a cardiovascular event may occur so infrequently that they are difficult or unethical to study directly. Biomarkers provide researchers with interim evidence about the safety and efficacy of interventions while more definitive clinical data are collected. In some cases, it may be preferable to use established biomarkers as surrogate endpoints to reduce the risk of harm to patients.[2] Though biomarkers have intrinsic characteristics, they also have contextual ones. Depending on how a biomarker is used, it could have a relationship to a number of other medical concepts as shown in Table 7.1.[1]

TABLE 7.1

Biomarker examples

Biomarker type	Example
Susceptibility to or the risk of developing a condition	• Gait characteristics (step-length during everyday walking) may be valid biomarkers to calculate fall risk in certain populations • Using a combination of genetic variants to predict the onset of age-related macular degeneration
Diagnosis or health status monitoring	• Presence or absence of P waves on an EKG trace obtained from a wearable/portable sensor as one of the inputs to a software algorithm to detect AFib that comes and goes (paroxysmal AFib) • Tremor detected in a limb at rest with a wrist-worn wearable may be one marker among several to help detect and monitor early Parkinson's disease

CONTINUED

TABLE 7.1 (CONTINUED)

Biomarker examples

Biomarker type	Example
Predicting whether an individual is more likely than others to experience a future change or clinical outcome	• A breast cancer patient's HER2 status can be a predictive biomarker when it is used to assess whether to treat with Herceptin. • The number of threshold-crossing events on an intrathoracic impedance signal measured by an implanted device may be a useful biomarker to enrich heart failure clinical studies with people more likely to experience clinical endpoints like hospitalization.[3,4]
Evaluating an individual's *prognosis*, or the likelihood that a disease recurs, progresses or is cured or that some other clinical event may happen in the future	• Using a composite mobility measure to predict future need for long-term care
Monitoring the molecular effects of an intervention	• Monitoring an antigen released by pancreatic cancer cells (CA 19-9) to judge a treatment's efficacy • Using a continuous glucose monitor to detect how a patient is reacting to insulin
Detecting a *safety* signal or adverse event	• Using a simple accelerometer or gyroscope for fall detection
Precisely quantifying the time course over which a dose of medicine has an effect on the body (its *pharmacodynamics*)	• Sweat chloride may be used when evaluating patients with cystic fibrosis, to assess response to cystic fibrosis transmembrane regulator-potentiating agents

AFib, atrial fibrillation; EKG, electrocardiogram; HER2, human epidermal growth factor receptor 2.

Although traditionally most biomarkers fall into the modalities of molecular, fluid or imaging categories, more digital biomarkers are being developed.[5] A digital biomarker could be any of the seven BEST biomarker types (see Figure 7.1).[5] The term digital refers to the method of collection as using sensors and computational tools, generally across multiple layers (e.g. a full stack) of hardware and software.[6]

Clinical outcome assessments

Clinical outcome assessments (COAs) are the instruments used to measure clinical outcomes, and include the instructions to participants, scoring models and protocols for administration (Figure 7.2).

There are currently four recognized types of COA (Table 7.2).[7]

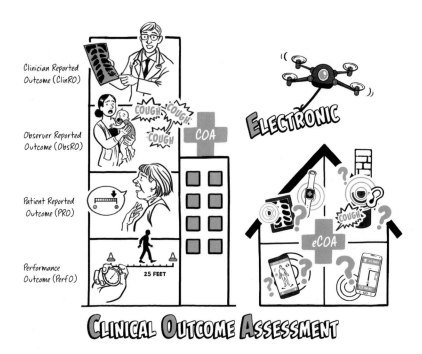

Figure 7.2 Clinical outcome assessment. Clinical outcome assessments (COAs) are the instruments used to measure clinical outcomes. The FDA recognizes four types: ClinRO, ObsRO, PRO and PerfO. If digitized, they are considered electronic (e)COAs.

TABLE 7.2

Clinical outcome assessment examples

COA	Example
ClinRO – requires clinical expertise	• 'Readings' are clearly defined results that are observed and reported in a dichotomous manner on the basis of clinicians' judgment, such as the presence or absence of clinician-identified radiographic vertebral fractures.[8] • 'Ratings' are categorical (either ordered or not) or continuous measures like those in Part III of the Unified Parkinson's Disease Rating Scale or the Brief Psychiatric Rating Scale in mental disorders.[8] • 'Clinician Global Assessments' (CGAs) are assessments based on a clinician's overall judgment like the 'clinician global impression' (CGI) or 'clinician global impression of change'.[8]
ObsRO – assessment of how patients feel or function in their daily lives made by a non-expert third party (e.g. spouse, caregiver, parent, sibling) Useful when the patient themselves may struggle to reliably assess their own symptoms and experiences (i.e. children or cognitively impaired)	• A parent's report of a child's vomiting episodes • A caregiver reporting a patient wincing through pain during activities when they cannot report this themselves

CONTINUED

TABLE 7.2 (CONTINUED)

Clinical outcome assessment examples

COA	Example
PRO – assessment about how patients feel or function in their daily lives where the information is reported by the patient themselves, without interpretation or modification by someone else	• Gastrointestinal Quality of Life instrument (GQLI) • European Organization for Research and Treatment of Cancer QLQ-C30 (EORTC QLQ-C30), a questionnaire that assesses the quality of life of patients with cancer • The Impact of Weight on Quality of Life (IWQOL-Lite) assesses obesity-specific quality of life measures
PerfO – assessment of a task(s) performed by a patient following instructions given by a healthcare professional Requires patient cooperation and motivation	• Timed 7.62 m (25 foot) walk test as a measure of gait speed • Severe Impairment Battery as a measure of cognitive function

ClinRO, clinician-reported outcome; COA, clinical outcome assessment; ObsRO, observer-reported outcome; PerfO, performance outcome; PRO, patient-reported outcome.

The industry generally makes a distinction between a digitally collected COA and a non-digital one (e.g. a paper questionnaire) by putting an 'e' for 'electronic' in front of the acronym (e.g. PRO [patient-reported outcome] to ePRO, COA to eCOA). Interestingly, though, the lines between technology-based assessments and questionnaires have become blurry. If a wearable device monitored your sleep overnight and then in the morning asked when you went to bed – was that evidence from a sensor or a questionnaire? As technologies continue to advance, there is increasing discussion around where digital measurement tools fit within this framework.

What if some of the human raters in the previous COA examples were replaced with technology? For example, a medically informed algorithm that processes movement data from a wearable to rate ataxia.

The possibility of a fifth COA to describe digital clinical outcome assessments, and specifically those measurements made using technology, was proposed during a summer 2018 Public Workshop at the FDA, though no firm next step was defined.[9]

Making human assessments digital

It takes far more work to make human assessments digital than to simply translate a paper questionnaire into an app and put an 'e' in front of the tool (e.g. PRO to ePRO). eCOAs have unique properties that offer new ways to measure outcomes. What matters is whether the concept being measured is directly meaningful to patients. Take, for example, multiple sclerosis (MS). 'Ability to go about my daily activities' is a meaningful aspect of health to MS patients.

A PRO (or even an ePRO) could measure a person's ability to perform activities of daily living through a self-reported survey. Self-reported measures require the person to reflect on and assess their own ability, leading to data that are meaningful to that individual, but potentially fraught with person-to-person variability, and subject to recall bias.

A PerfO (performance outcome) might measure the amount of time it takes a person to walk 25 m. This is easy to measure and may be correlated with the capacity to perform typical daily activities. This approach has the benefit of not relying on patient recall, but it is an imperfect measure of the real outcome of interest – the ability to perform daily living tasks in a natural environment.

A multimodal product may continuously and passively assess total daily activity (mins), average daily walking speed (m/s), and number of sit-stand transitions per day (n). This is a much, much closer approximation of the meaningful aspect of health than the PerfO, or even the 'ePerfO', but is not accompanied by the bias and subjectivity of the PRO or ePRO.

Composite measures. We can also combine multimodal data from sensors, questionnaires and other clinical data (e.g. lab test, genomic tests) to create composite measures or 'complex biomarkers'.[7]

A composite measure consists of several individual measures that are combined to reach a single interpretive readout. For example, you could use sensor, keyboard, voice and speech data from a smartphone to construct a composite measure for cognition, and augment that measure over time with genetic data to make it more multimodal.[10]

The need for a human intermediary. Over time, a useful distinction between metric types will be whether the measurement required action by a human intermediary to gather the data (Figure 7.3). At the passive end of the spectrum, human participation is minimal and sensors simply capture data as individuals engage in daily activities like eating and sleeping. At the active end of the spectrum, more action by the intermediary is required. This could include a patient entering information into an electronic sleep diary or performing a task like a cognitive test. Hybrids of these two measures that use multimodal assessments and combine active and passive measures will also be valuable. An example is using actigraphy to passively measure when an individual fell asleep, coupled with an ePRO asking the individual to self-report the time.

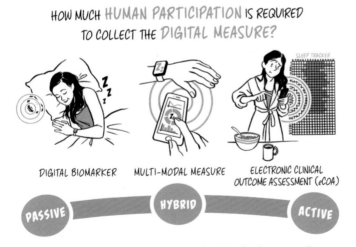

HOW MUCH HUMAN PARTICIPATION IS REQUIRED TO COLLECT THE DIGITAL MEASURE?

DIGITAL BIOMARKER   MULTI-MODAL MEASURE   ELECTRONIC CLINICAL OUTCOME ASSESSMENT (eCOA)

PASSIVE   HYBRID   ACTIVE

Figure 7.3 Human participation. Connected technologies can collect physiological and behavioral data. Some do so passively via sensors, while others (like sleep tracker surveys) may be more active in nature. Some are a hybrid where they will track some metrics algorithmically and then ask for confirmation.

Key points – digital biomarkers and clinical outcomes

- 'Effective, unambiguous communication is essential for efficient translation of promising scientific discoveries into approved medical products' (US Food and Drug Administration, BEST framework). Today, many key terms and definitions have been used inconsistently, and this ambiguity makes it difficult to evaluate products and evidence.

- For many measurements, it can be helpful to think about whether the data were collected actively through human intervention (e.g. a clinician observing the patient, or a patient filling in a diary) or passively through a sensor.

- Most high-quality data sources will likely be 'multimodal', meaning that the data will come from multiple sensors.

- Developing a common set of language around biomarkers, measurements, outcomes and other terms will streamline premarket discussions between regulators and industry, and also postmarket with patients and providers. The authors defined a first draft set of definitions, which we expect and hope will evolve as technologies and applications develop over time.

- If someone uses a term you don't know in a conversation, best practice is to ask the person to clarify what they mean. Many terms are still in early development and have loose definitions.

References

1. FDA-NIH Biomarker Working Group. Glossary. In: *BEST (Biomarkers, EndpointS, and other Tools) Resource*, 2018. www.ncbi.nlm.nih.gov/books/NBK338448/, last accessed 31 July 2019.

2. Strimbu K, Tavel JA. What are biomarkers? *Curr Opin HIV AIDS* 2010;5: 463–6.

3. Kramer F, Dinh W. Molecular and digital biomarker supported decision making in clinical studies in cardiovascular indications. *Arch Pharm* 2016;349:399–409.

4. Miyoshi A, Nishii N, Kubo M et al. An improved algorithm calculated from intrathoracic impedance can precisely diagnose preclinical heart failure events: Sub-analysis of a multicenter MOMOTARO (Monitoring and Management of OptiVol Alert to Reduce Heart Failure Hospitalization) trial study. *J Cardiol* 2017;70:425–31.

5. Coravos A, Khozin S, Mandl KD. Developing and adopting safe and effective digital biomarkers to improve patient outcomes. *npj Digit Med* 2019;2:14.

6. Califf RM. Biomarker definitions and their applications. *Exp Biol Med* 2018;243:213–21.

7. FDA-NIH Biomarker Working Group. *BEST (Biomarkers, EndpointS, and other Tools) Resource*, 2016. www.ncbi.nlm.nih.gov/books/NBK326791/, last accessed 31 July 2019.

8. Powers III JH, Patrick DL, Walton MK et al. Clinician-reported outcome assessments of treatment benefit: report of the ISPOR Clinical Outcome Assessment Emerging Good Practices Task Force. *Value Health* 2017; 20:2–14.

9. US Food and Drug Administration. *FDA Public Workshop: 2018 Clinical Outcome Assessments in Cancer Clinical Trials*, 2018. www.fda.gov/newsevents/meetingsconferences workshops/ucm602540.htm, last accessed 31 July 2019.

10. Insel TR. Digital phenotyping: technology for a new science of behavior. *JAMA* 2017;318:1215–16.

8   Measurement in clinical trials

The goal of any trial is to determine both the safety and efficacy of a new medical product. Measures within the trial process must demonstrate the product's safety and efficacy to regulators before it is allowed to be labeled and marketed for use by patients.

However, measurement in clinical trials does not only inform regulatory decision-making. Early in the development of a new drug or novel medical device, a company will make business decisions about whether to advance its new product for further testing. Early intelligence is extremely valuable to biopharma companies, which face a US$2 million revenue opportunity per day the drug is on the market (or not).[1] Digital measures allow for the collection of data outside of the clinic, providing a more continuous stream of data points on whether the drug or device is working or not.

Additionally, measurement data from clinical trials inform reimbursement decisions, which impacts the value of the market. In countries like the US that depend on third-party (e.g. non-government) payers, insurance companies need evidence to decide *whether* to reimburse the manufacturer for their approved product and *at what price*. In countries with a single-payer system, often the decision about pricing coincides with the regulatory approvals process.

Trial success is not correlated with number of measures. It is much more important to select the *right* measures – those that are the most informative regarding the product's safety and efficacy – rather than the *most* measures. In fact, medical product manufacturers, regulators, patients and ethics review boards all worry about burdening participants with excessive tasks, activities and technologies. The ability of a measure to effectively and accurately operate in the wild (e.g. out of a patient's home and across many geographies and languages) is also a concern. Medical product manufacturers are often reluctant to assume even more risk – not just in their new product but also in a novel measure – without a substantial body of evidence.

Decisions regarding the inclusion of digital measurement tools in clinical trials are complex, affect many stakeholders and require extensive consideration of factors related to the clinical implications of the measure itself. Additionally, the operational aspects of the measure and the potential effects on the trial design and participants need to be considered (Figure 8.1).

Changing clinical trials

Traditional clinical trials collect snippets of data when a participant visits the study site and represent a tiny snapshot of patients' lived experience with a disease or condition. Yet researchers, industry sponsors and regulators rely on this limited information to make life-or-death decisions and multibillion-dollar investments.

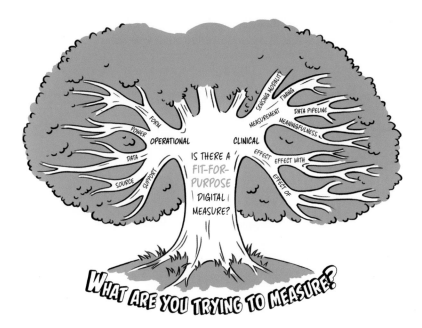

Figure 8.1 Fit-for-purpose digital measure decision tree. Decisions about what to measure in a clinical trial are rooted in the research question being posed. Whether a fit-for-purpose digital measure exists to help to answer that question depends on both clinical and operational considerations that involve many stakeholders.

Digital measurements will convert that snapshot into a movie, with the ability to collect near continuous data outside the physical confines of the clinical environment, such as in a person's home, using connected products, including smartphones, wearables, implantables and ingestible devices and sensors.

Decentralized clinical trials. Digital tools enable new forms of research such as decentralized clinical trials (DCTs), which are conducted outside of the clinic to capture data about a study participant in their day-to-day life (Figure 8.2).

DCTs have a number of potential benefits, including faster participant recruitment, improved participant retention in the trial, greater control and convenience for participants, increased diversity (e.g. because it is easier to enroll in the first place) and trial results that are more generalizable.[2,3]

DCTs offer a way to make better-informed decisions about the efficacy of new therapies. More sensitive, objective measures from

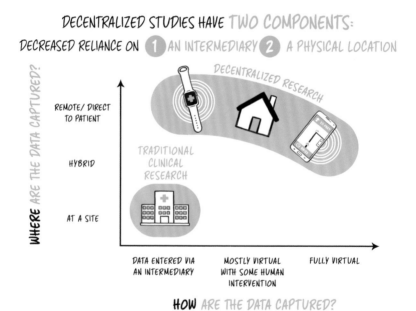

Figure 8.2 Decentralized clinical trials. There are two components to consider to determine the level of decentralization in a clinical trial: whether the data are captured at a site or near the patient (e.g. location), and how the data are captured (e.g. manually or digitally).

digital technologies coupled with a greater density of information – continuously sampling multiple times a day, not just once a quarter – will help the industry fail faster and win more efficiently.

Two features of data collection determine how 'decentralized' a clinical trial is:[4] where and how the data are collected.

Where are data collected? In traditional clinical trials, drugs, devices and therapies are administered in a clinic or research hospital. In newer direct-to-patient or remote trials, participant data are collected in the home or in the study participant's natural environment.

How are the data collected? In the past, most data were collected via an intermediary – someone from the team would record information in a custom software system and/or case report form. As digital tools advance, we can collect more endpoint-supporting data at home via digital surveys and sensors, and study teams can 'visit' patients at home via telemedicine conference calls. This means that more of the data are participant-generated and collected 'virtually', without an intermediary.

In context. A doctor who remote teleconferences with a patient would be conducting a 'remote trial', but they might collect the data manually through a survey, so the study would not be considered a 'virtual trial'. In contrast, a study team might collect all the data passively from a smartwatch in a clinic, and this study would be a 'virtual trial' from a data collection perspective, but not a 'remote trial' because the patient is in a centralized location.

Notably, the industry has not yet settled on language around these types of trials, which is not unexpected. As a new field emerges, so does a new vocabulary. Historically, some researchers, primarily behavioral scientists, have referred to this type of study as a community-based clinical trial (CBCT) as a clinic may not be involved in the intervention being tested.[5] The US Food and Drug Administration (FDA) has been using the term DCT more often in the past few years to describe trials taking place at home or in the community.[6]

What are real-world data?
Real world is a term that is important to define as it is often misused. The regulatory definition of real-world data is the data collected outside of a traditional clinical study, such as a randomized controlled

trial (RCT).[7] These data sources include electronic health records (EHRs), claims and billing activities,
product and disease registries, patient-generated data including in home-use settings, and data gathered from other sources that can inform on health status, such as mobile technologies.[7]

Real-world evidence is the evidence derived from real-world data.[8] In the context of a traditional RCT, if study participants contribute to some measurements at home, such as pain measurement via an electronic patient-reported outcome (ePRO) or step count from a wearable sensor, many often mistakenly believe this would constitute real-world data. However, these measures would not constitute real-world data because the participants have been preselected for study entry by the inclusion and exclusion criteria of a given trial. They do not represent the overall population in a certain indication. Therefore, when working with clinical research, it is important to focus on the benefits of health-related data collected in natural settings – which may not be classified as 'real world' by a strict regulatory definition.

Key points – measurement in clinical trials

- Decentralized clinical trials (DCTs), which are conducted in a study participant's home using digital tools, offer a way to make better-informed decisions about the efficacy of new therapies.
- DCTs are characterized by two core questions: where are the data collected (e.g. how remote is the study?) and how are the data collected (e.g. how virtual is the study? How much of the data is collected using digital tools versus needing human interaction?)?
- DCTs have a number of potential benefits, including faster participant recruitment, improved participant retention in the trial, greater control and convenience for participants and increased diversity and inclusion (e.g. because it is easier to enroll in the first place).
- Digital measurement tools collect real-world data only when used outside of a clinical trial. When data from these tools are collected as part of a clinical trial protocol, they are collecting data during activities of daily living. But it is incorrect to call these data 'real-world data' as this term has a specific regulatory meaning.

References

1. Paul SM, Mytelka DS, Dunwiddie CT et al. How to improve R&D productivity: the pharmaceutical industry's grand challenge. *Nat Rev Drug Discov* 2010;9:203–14.

2. Khozin S, Coravos A. Decentralized trials in the age of real-world evidence and inclusivity in clinical investigations. *Clin Pharmacol Ther* 2019;106:25–7.

3. Clinical Trials Transformation Initiative. *Project: Decentralized Clinical Trials*, 2016. www.ctti-clinicaltrials.org/projects/decentralized-clinical-trials, last accessed 31 July 2019.

4. Coravos A. Decentralized clinical trials. *Elektra Labs Blog*, 2018. https://medium.com/elektra-labs/decentralized-clinical-trials-f12fffb72610, last accessed 31 July 2019.

5. King AC, Haskell WL, Taylor CB et al. Group- vs home-based exercise training in healthy older men and women. A community-based clinical trial. *JAMA* 1991;266:1535–42.

6. Gottlieb S (US Food and Drug Administration). *Breaking Down Barriers Between Clinical Trials and Clinical Care: Incorporating Real World Evidence into Regulatory Decision Making* [speech], 2019.www.fda.gov/NewsEvents/Speeches/ucm629942.htm, last accessed 31 July 2019.

7. US Food and Drug Administration. *Real-World Evidence*, 2019. www.fda.gov/scienceresearch/specialtopics/realworldevidence/default.htm, last accessed 31 July 2019.

8. Makady A, de Boer A, Hillege H et al. on behalf of GetReal Work Package 1. What is real-world data? A review of definitions based on literature and stakeholder interviews. *Value Health* 2017;20:858–65.

9 Verification and validation

How do I assure myself and others that my digital measurement tool generates good, trustworthy data (Figure 9.1)? Verification and validation (V&V) are two processes that, together, indicate whether a digital measurement tool is fit for purpose.

Understanding the processes

Once you have arrived at a construct to measure and you have some ideas about the way a digital tool could be used to measure it, there are a number of ways to assure yourself and others that the tool generates high-quality, meaningful and trustworthy data. Verification and validation are terms that are probably familiar to you if you come from an engineering or product development background. They apply to digital medicine, too.

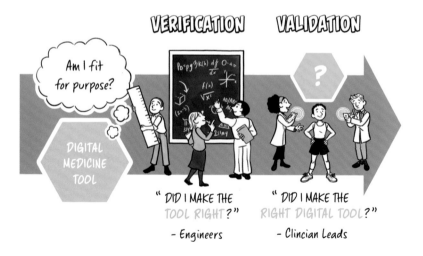

Figure 9.1 Verification and validation.

Verification is the assessment of sensor accuracy (which describes the agreement between the measurement made by a single sensor versus a ground truth), precision (which describes the agreement between multiple measurements made by a single sensor back-to-back), consistency (which describes the agreement between multiple measurements made by a single sensor over longer time periods) and/or uniformity (which describes the agreement across measurements made by multiple sensors simultaneously). A sensor that is accurate, precise, consistent and uniform will 'give the right answer every time'.

By undertaking verification assessments, the investigator can also be assured that the relevant firmware/software that generates processed data is also accurate, precise, consistent and uniform.[1] Verification answers the question 'did I make the tool right?' Verification is an *engineering assessment*, and it is entirely separate from data collection from humans.

Validation is the process of ensuring that the digital measurement tool is meeting its intended use by generating objective data that accurately represent the concept of interest – the specific way in which the patient feels, functions or survives – that it purports to be measuring. Validation answers the question 'did I build the right tool?' The concept of validation can be broken down as follows.

Analytic validation. Is the algorithm processing the data to report the measurement of interest? For example, is the algorithm accurately processing raw accelerometry data to calculate gait speed in a particular patient population?

Clinical validation. Is the measurement of interest reflecting the concept of interest – the specific way in which the patient feels, functions or survives? For example, is gait speed a meaningful measure that reflects how a particular patient population feels, functions or survives?

To answer whether the technology is measuring what it is intended to measure (clinical validation) and is correct (analytic validation), developers should work with researchers to ensure that validation studies are well designed.

Separating the sensor and the measure is the most important concept to remember when considering V&V. All sensors can be boiled down to the physical construct that is measured, such as acceleration, temperature or pressure.

The process of *verification* evaluates the capture and transference of a sensor-generated signal into collected data. As verification studies typically happen at the bench without human subjects, they do not usually require ethics committee review. *Validation* almost always involves human subject testing; it is the process of ensuring that the output data from the technology are accurate against a gold standard (analytic validation) and an appropriate reflection of the clinical concept of interest (clinical validation). Answering the latter will often involve testing the technology with human participants, which may require an ethics committee review before testing (see chapter 5).

Clinical validation has multiple dimensions. We will not go into all of them here, but one example is whether a change in your new measurement is regarded as meaningful by people with the disease. Do the results generated by the tool capture all aspects of the concept you are measuring? Do changes to measurement values predict certain clinical outcomes down the road? Does the measurement respond to an intervention that is well understood to have an effect on the property you are measuring in that population? Can the measure correctly identify those patients with and without the condition (sensitivity and specificity)? Likewise, does that property remain unchanged in circumstances when it should not change (e.g. in a different population or when there is no intervention)? Of particular note in the realm of digital medicine is the reliance on computational algorithms, the performance of which can improve over time given access to more representative datasets (see chapter 1). The regulatory framework to deal with such systems is under active development at the US Food and Drug Administration (FDA).[2]

Often, researchers will ask how a novel digital measure compares with a gold-standard assessment. We believe 'gold standard' is often a misnomer because many gold standards are not necessarily high-quality measures. If the most widely used existing measurement is suboptimal, more appropriate terms include legacy standard, where a new and better measurement has been developed, or current standard, in cases where the standard is acknowledged to be inadequate but no alternative yet exists.

For example, the legacy assessment in Duchenne's muscular dystrophy (DMD) is the 6-minute walk test. This is a poor endpoint for a number of reasons. First, it does not apply to the roughly 60% of that patient population who are confined to a wheelchair and cannot participate in a walk test.

Second, DMD trial participants typically range in age from 7 years (though this has been noted to be lowering in recent years) to mid-teens, so bias may be introduced in a number of directions; in some cases owing to issues of diminished patient volition and in others through coaching or gaming by parents of young participants. These biases may lead to noise that obscures the endpoint.

Finally, many consider that the 6-minute walk test fails to demonstrate strong ecological validity, that is, it is a poor measure of how test performance predicts behaviors in real-world settings. Stellmann et al.[3] offer an excellent exploration of the ecological validity of mobility outcomes, including the 6-minute walk test, in multiple sclerosis and consider the opportunities for digital tools to improve these measures.

Regardless of the quality of a legacy standard, it is unlikely that a digital measurement will agree perfectly with the existing standard. In fact, for this reason, digital measures garner a lot of excitement: they may turn out to be more sensitive than traditional measures or be capable of measuring something researchers have never been able to measure before. Traditional measurements provide only a tiny snapshot of information about a patient's experience of their disease, and they are also fraught with confounders such as white coat syndrome, where a patient's feeling of anxiety in a medical environment results in an abnormally high reading when assessing blood pressure.[4]

In other instances, a digital assessment may measure an aspect of disease that has been inaccessible with traditional measures. For the DMD example, a more inclusive digital measurement could be of upper limb mobility, which can be applied to a much broader population of DMD patients. However, there would be little utility in trying to tether this new digital measure against the legacy standard of a 6-minute walk test.

To summarize simply, if the test can be performed by a good engineer or physicist who flunked biology, then it is verification. If it requires medical knowledge, it is validation.

When is something 'validated' enough?

The answer depends on the specific application. Tools need to be fit for purpose. The level of validation associated with a medical product development tool should be sufficient to support its context of use, a regulatory term that refers to a description of how the tool is used and where it is applied.[5]

The Clinical Trials Transformation Initiative (CTTI), a public private partnership co-founded by Duke University and the FDA, has developed comprehensive recommendations and resources on developing digital measurement tools for use as clinical trial endpoints.[6] This may be a valuable resource for anyone looking to understand the body of evidence that is required to support the use of a digital medicine tool in a clinical trial.

Increasing overlap between clinical research and care

Historically, measures that support research (endpoints) and care (outcomes) were siloed. But that is changing: many clinically validated endpoints used in research will likely transition into clinical care. A number of companies are working toward a universal vision of human digital measurement across the continuum of research and clinical care. Clinical research provides a practical approach by which we can link (or validate) everyday behaviors and outcomes. Companies that develop digital biomarkers validate these tools through clinical research as a first step toward what may eventually become a validated digital diagnostic or a digital therapeutic.

Similarly, a number of big tech companies are also developing digital measures for clinical settings. In 2018, the FDA cleared a 'software as a medical device' (SaMD) for the Apple Watch, which can determine the presence of atrial fibrillation, an abnormal heart condition. This clearance provides a regulatory pathway for companies to create more advanced diagnostics and interventions for the patient, at home, decentralized.

There is crossover in use between research and routine care, such as the safety monitoring of trial participants during the course of a clinical study. However, even in such crossover cases, the clinical trial environment is by its nature more structured and controlled than the variety of settings and scenarios where clinical medicine is practiced.

Key points – verification and validation

- Verification evaluates the capture and transference of a sensor-generated signal into collected data. The goal of verification testing is to ensure that the sensor is accurate, precise, consistent and uniform. This usually does not require human subjects.
- Validation ensures that the technology is measuring what it is intended to measure. It almost always requires human subjects. Validation comprises two types of testing:
  - Analytic validation: does the device process the raw data to produce the measure of interest (e.g. convert raw accelerometry data to gait speed in a particular patient population)?
  - Clinical validation: do changes to the measure of interest predict future clinical outcomes (e.g. is gait speed a marker of disease progression)?
- The level of validation associated with a digital measure should be sufficient to support its context of use, a regulatory term that refers to a description of how the tool is used and where it is applied.
- There is increasing overlap between clinical research and care. Digital biomarkers may initially be validated in the context of clinical research, and eventually transition to a validated digital diagnostic or a digital therapeutic.

References

1. Clinical Trials Transformation Initiative. *Figure 2. Data Processes and Information to Provide to FDA.* www.ctti-clinicaltrials.org/sites/www.ctti-clinicaltrials.org/files/figure-2-data-process-fda-submission.pdf, last accessed 31 July 2019.

2. US Food and Drug Administration. *Proposed Regulatory Framework for Modifications to Artificial Intelligence/Machine Learning (AI/ML)-Based Software as a Medical Device (SaMD).* www.fda.gov/downloads/MedicalDevices/DigitalHealth/SoftwareasaMedicalDevice/UCM635052.pdf, last accessed 31 July 2019.

3. Stellmann JP, Neuhaus A, Götze N et al. Ecological validity of walking capacity tests in multiple sclerosis. *PLoS One* 2015;10:e0123822.

4. Banegas JR, Ruilope LM, de la Sierra A et al. Relationship between clinic and ambulatory blood-pressure measurements and mortality. *N Engl J Med* 2018; 378:1509–20.

5. Izmailova ES, Wagner JA, Perakslis ED. Wearable devices in clinical trials: hype and hypothesis. *Clin Pharmacol Ther* 2018;104:42–52.

6. Clinical Trials Transformation Initiative. *Developing Novel Endpoints Generated by Mobile Technology for Use in Clinical Trials,* 2017. www.ctti-clinicaltrials.org/briefing-room/recommendations/developing-novel-endpoints-generated-mobile-technology-use-clinical, last accessed 31 July 2019.

10 The future of digital medicine

The field of digital medicine is hitting an inflection point. More granular and, potentially, high-quality data can now be collected and transmitted in near real time. These data are now available to be used for measurement and in health interventions – clearly the time is now for shaping this future healthcare model. There are ontologies, frameworks and decision-support tools that we need to develop to ensure that the advent of digital medicine leads to a better healthcare system. Clarifying language and establishing a standard lexicon will advance the field faster, together and with more trust. This book was written to provide the foundational basis, with a goal of increasing understanding among those involved in shaping the nascent field of digital medicine. Recognizing that the field will evolve over time, we view this edition as a first stake in the ground.

Our community faces challenging decisions – particularly ethical ones around surveillance, convenience, personalization and privacy – and it is important to remember that all systems are first built by humans who design the incentives. Let us build an intentional future that we want to live in, and not an accidental one. We must ensure that we adopt healthcare technologies that are worthy of the trust we place in them.[1]

The Digital Medicine Society (DiMe) exists to advance digital medicine to optimize human health. We are the professional home for professionals at the intersection of the global healthcare and technology communities, supporting them in developing digital medicine through interdisciplinary collaboration, research, teaching, and the promotion of best practices. If you are passionate about building an intentional future for digital medicine, join us, and build it with us. www.dimesociety.org/index.php/membership

Key points – the future of digital medicine

- Clarifying language and establishing a standard lexicon will advance the field faster, together and with more trust.
- Together, we are designing the incentives that will guide challenging decisions around surveillance, convenience, personalization and privacy.
- Collectively, we are responsible for ensuring that digital medicine tools are worthy of the trust we place in them.

Reference

1. I Am The Cavalry. *I Am The Cavalry Cyber Safety Outreach.* www.iamthecavalry.org, last accessed 31 July 2019.

Useful resources

Organizations

CORE Platform
An interactive collaboration platform for researchers conducting digital health research and for institutional review boards charged with reviewing this research: https://thecore-platform.ucsd.edu/

Clinical Trials Transformation Initiative
A collaboration that includes government agencies, industry representatives, patient advocacy groups, professional societies, investigator groups and academic institutions that aims to develop and drive the adoption of practices to improve the quality and efficiency of clinical trials: www.ctti-clinicaltrials.org

Digital Medicine Society (DiMe)
The professional society for the digital medicine community. Together, we drive scientific progress and broad acceptance of digital medicine to enhance public health: www.dimesociety.org/

I Am The Cavalry
An organization working to ensure that technologies are worthy of the trust we place in them: www.iamthecavalry.org

ReCODE Health
The Research Center for Optimal Digital Ethics in Health at University of California, San Diego, California, USA, supports researchers, developers, participants and institutions involved with digital health research: https://recode.health

Sage Bionetworks
A non-profit biomedical research and technology development organization that develops and applies open practices to data-driven research for the advancement of human health: https://sagebionetworks.org

The Digital Therapeutics Alliance
A non-profit trade association of industry leaders and stakeholders with a mission to 'broaden the understanding, adoption, and integration of clinically validated digital therapeutics into healthcare through education, advocacy, and research': www.dtxalliance.org/about-dta/

Guidance and tools
FDA-NIH Biomarker Working Group. BEST (Biomarkers, EndpointS, and other Tools) Resource, 2016. www.ncbi.nlm.nih.gov/books/NBK326791/, last accessed 31 July 2019.

US Food and Drug Administration. Guidances with Digital Health Content: www.fda.gov/medical-devices/digital-health/guidances-digital-health-content

Publications
Agboola SO, Bates DW, Kvedar JC. Digital health and patient safety. *JAMA* 2016;315:1697–8.

Chang SM, Matchar DB, Smetana GW et al., eds. *Methods Guide for Medical Test Reviews*. Rockville: Agency for Healthcare Research and Quality; 2012. www.ncbi.nlm.nih.gov/books/NBK98241/

Coravos A, Khozin S, Mandl KD. Developing and adopting safe and effective digital biomarkers to improve patient outcomes. *npj Digital Medicine* 2019;2:14.

Goldsack J. Laying the foundation: defining digital medicine. DiMe, 2019. https://medium.com/digital-medicine-society-dime/laying-the-foundation-defining-digital-medicine-49ab7b6ab6ef, last accessed 21 August 2019.

International Medical Device Regulators Forum. Software as a Medical Device (SaMD) [work complete – historical reference]. www.imdrf.org/workitems/wi-samd.asp, last accessed 31 July 2019.

Manta C. Digital medicine standards 101. DiMe, 2019. https://medium.com/digital-medicine-society-dime/standards-for-digital-medicine-1a44b743c347, last accessed 25 September 2019.

Nebeker C, Bartlett Ellis RJ, Torous J. Development of a decision-making checklist tool to support technology selection in digital health research. *Transl Behav Med* 2019;ibz074.

Steinhubl SR, Topol EJ. Digital medicine, on its way to being just plain medicine. *npj Digit Med* 2018:20175.

US Food and Drug Administration. *The FDA's Role in Medical Device Cybersecurity: Dispelling Myths and Understanding Facts*, 2017. www.fda.gov/media/103696/download, last accessed 21 August 2019.

Wang T, Azad T, Rajan R. The emerging influence of digital biomarkers on healthcare. *Rock Health*. https://rockhealth.com/reports/the-emerging-influence-of-digital-biomarkers-on-healthcare/, last accessed 24 September 2019.

Woods B, Coravos A, Corman JD. The case for a Hippocratic oath for connected medical devices: viewpoint. *J Med Internet Res* 2019;21:e12568.

Zimmerman N. Lessons learned implementing Apple ResearchKit for a study at Mount Sinai. DiMe, 2019. https://medium.com/digital-medicine-society-dime/lessons-learned-implementing-apple-researchkit-for-a-study-at-mount-sinai-1b962a04ad83, last accessed 21 August 2019.

Journals
Digital Biomarkers: www.karger.com/Journal/Home/271954

npj Digital Medicine: www.nature.com/npjdigitalmed/

Index